T0230491

Health Promotion with Adolescent Boys
and Young Men of Colour

James A. Smith • Daphne C. Watkins
Derek M. Griffith

Editors

Health Promotion with Adolescent Boys and Young Men of Colour

Global Strategies for Advancing Research, Policy, and Practice in Context

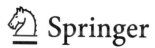 Springer

Editors
James A. Smith
Rural and Remote Health
College of Medicine and Public Health
Flinders University
Darwin, NT, Australia

Daphne C. Watkins
School of Social Work
University of Michigan–Ann Arbor
Ann Arbor, MI, USA

Derek M. Griffith
Department of Health Management
and Policy
School of Health
Center for Men's Health Equity
Racial Justice Institute
Georgetown University
Washington, DC, USA

ISBN 978-3-031-22176-7   ISBN 978-3-031-22174-3   (eBook)
https://doi.org/10.1007/978-3-031-22174-3

This Springer imprint is published by the registered company Springer Nature Switzerland AG
The registered company address is: Gewerbestrasse 11, 6330 Cham, Switzerland

Preface

Over the past few years, there has been a rapid expansion of global commentary relating to men's health equity (Griffith et al., 2019; Baker, 2020; Griffith, 2020; Smith et al., 2020; Smith et al., 2020). It has provided a new, and arguably more helpful, gender-health lens from which to view the health and social inequities experienced by marginalised and vulnerable groups of boys and men (Griffith et al., 2019; Griffith, 2020; Smith et al., 2020). Indeed, it has enabled a more nuanced discourse about the health and well-being of specific sub-populations of men to emerge, including that relating to men of colour (Jones et al., 2012; Griffith et al., 2019; Smith et al., 2019, 2021). Most recently, there has been increased interest in the health inequities experienced by *adolescent boys* and *young* men of colour (Cunningham & White, 2019; Smith et al., 2021). This book helps to expand on this discussion.

Our primary aim, in this book, is to explore what the health promotion community has done, and can continue to do, to reduce the health and social inequities facing boys and young men of colour across the globe. While there are pockets of health promotion innovation strategies targeting boys and young men of colour, these strategies are typically poorly funded, time-bound, and seldom scaled to a level to meet population health needs (Smith et al., 2021).

Why Write a Book About Health Promotion and Young Men of Colour?

As men's health promotion scholars, we know that there is a paucity of evidence about the most promising health-promotion strategies to improve the health and well-being of boys and young men (Armstrong & Cohall, 2011). This is exacerbated further when it comes to boys and young men of colour (Smith et al., 2021). The existing scholarship is diffuse, often lacks research and evaluative rigour, and appears more abundant in grey literature than peer-reviewed scholarship. This impedes the planning and implementation of robust evidence-based health promotion strategies targeting boys and young men of colour. We subsequently call for more gender-sensitive, culturally responsive, and age-appropriate health promotion action to serve this highly marginalised population (Smith et al., 2020).

What Do You Need to Know Before Reading This Book?

There are a few important insights to share before you read this book.

First, young men of colour are not a homogenous group. Recognising the heterogeneity among this population is critical for understanding the potential health promotion actions that can follow. This edited collection deliberately reflects geographical, cultural, and social diversity among young men of colour. It includes contributions from Australia, Canada, New Zealand, the United States, and the Pacific Islands. It draws on research and interventions with African American, Aboriginal and Torres Strait Islander, Maori, Native American, and other First Nations young men. Yet, we recognise that this contribution only paints a partial picture. Other marginalised groups of boys and young men of colour, such as those from Latinx and Asian backgrounds, are equally deserving of such attention, but are under-represented in this book. Nevertheless, we trust this collection provides the impetus for a broader and more diverse array of voices to emerge over the longer term. As such, we encourage people working in these spaces to promote and share their learnings with others.

Second, the health promotion work happening with boys and young men of colour spans research, policy, and practice settings. All of these domains are reflected in one way or another throughout this book. Indeed, some chapters focus on men's health promotion research and preferentially offer guidance about promising health promotion interventions. In contrast, other chapters provide evaluative evidence about implementing health promotion programs targeting boys and young men of colour. These contributions are equally important. We urge our readers to engage with this breadth of perspectives, as there are different lessons in each chapter that can influence future health promotion research, policy, and practice in this field.

Third, it was evident from the chapters submitted for this book that there has been a groundswell in health promotion research and programs with an explicit mental health or social and emotional well-being orientation. This is an important observation in advancing health promotion efforts with boys and young men of colour, and is consistent with other recent scholarship on this topic (Watkins, 2019). In particular, it demonstrates there is room to incorporate more progressive forms of masculinity in the way mental health promotion strategies are developed with boys and young men of colour. This marks a significant step forward in health promotion scholarship and practice. We are pleased there are multiple examples of this throughout the book, which offer new insights about more explicit strengths-based approaches to health promotion with boys and young men of colour.

Finally, it is difficult to pull together such diverse chapters into a cohesive whole. We were initially tempted to edit chapters in a way that standardised their format and tone. After much consideration, we decided not to edit the chapters in this way. It was important that we presented the chapters authentically, in the way the authors and the communities they work with had intended. Each chapter tells a unique story. We consider this is a reflection of the current field of scholarship focused on health promotion and young men of colour. This diversity should be celebrated, not homogenised. We trust our readers will embrace this intent and glean from this new and emerging evidence base. Please enjoy the read ahead.

Darwin, NT, Australia   James A. Smith
Ann Arbor, MI, USA   Daphne C. Watkins
Washington, DC, USA   Derek M. Griffith

References

Armstrong, B. & Cohall, A. (2011). Health promotion with adolescent and young adult males: An empowerment approach. In A. Cohall & M. Resnick (Eds.), *Advances in Health Promotion for Adolescents and Young Adults - Adolescent Medicine: State of the Art Reviews*. Chicago: American Academy of Pediatrics.

Baker P. (2020). *From the Margins to the Mainstream: Next Steps. Achieving the Inclusion of Men's Health in Policy*. Global Action on Men's Health, London (UK).

Cunningham, M. & White, A. (2019). Young adulthood and health disparities in African American males. In D. M. Griffith, M. A. Bruce & R. J. Thorpe, Jr. (Eds.), *Men's Health Equity: A Handbook* (p. 57–71). New York: Routledge.

Griffith, D. M. (2020). Promoting men's health equity. *American Journal of Men's Health. 14*(6), 1–7.

Griffith, D. M., Bruce, M. A. & Thorpe, Jr., R. J. (2019). Introduction. In D. M. Griffith, M. A. Bruce & R. J. Thorpe, Jr. (Eds.), *Men's Health Equity: A Handbook* (p. 3–9). New York, Routledge.

Jones, D., Crump, A. & Lloyd, J. (2012). Health disparities in boys and men of color. *American Journal of Public Health, 102*(S2), S170–S172.

Smith, J., Drummond, M., Adams, M., Bonson, J. & Christie, B. (2019). Understanding men's health inequities in Australia (p. 498–509). In D. M. Griffith, M. A. Bruce & R. J. Thorpe, Jr. (Eds.), *Men's Health Equity: A Handbook* (p. 498–509). New York, Routledge.

Smith, J., Griffith, D.M., White, A., Baker, P., Watkins, D., Drummond, M. & Semlow, A. (2020). COVID-19, equity and men's health: Using evidence to inform future public health policy, practice and research responses in pandemics. *International Journal of Men's Social and Community Health, 3*(1), e48–e64.

Smith, J., Watkins, D. & Griffith, D. M. (2020). Equity, gender, and health: New directions for global men's health promotion. *Health Promotion Journal of Australia, 31*(2), 161–165.

Smith, J., Watkins, D. & Griffith, D. M. (2021). Reducing health inequities facing boys and young black men in the US. *Health Promotion International, 36*(5), 1508–1515.

Smith, J., Watkins, D., Griffith, D. M., Richardson, N. & Adams, M. (2020). Strengthening policy commitments to equity and men's health. *International Journal of Men's Social and Community Health, 3*(3), e9–e10.

Watkins, D. (2019). A light on the path to and promise for Black men's mental health. *Men and Masculinities, 22*(5), 917–920.

Acknowledgements

The editors would like to acknowledge the Australian-American Fulbright Commission for supporting Professor Smith to visit the United States of America throughout 2020. This provided an opportunity for Professor Smith, Professor Watkins, and Professor Griffith to meet and work collaboratively on the development of this book. Despite the various interruptions caused by COVID-19, we trust this book will leave a lasting legacy that will benefit boys and young men of colour globally.

We would like to extend our thanks and appreciation to Dr. Liz Adamson, Dr. Daile Rung, and Mr. Jahdai Vigona from the Freemasons Centre for Male Health and Wellbeing – Northern Territory for assisting with a variety of administrative tasks during the preparation of the book.

We would also like to thank Leslie Castro-Woodhouse, Owner and Principal of Origami Editorial, for copyediting the chapters prior to publication.

We would like to thank all of the book chapter authors. Your contributions and unique insights are critical for advancing the field of health promotion with young men of colour.

Thanks also to Janet Kim at Springer for your patience as we navigated the development of the book.

Contents

About the Editors

James A. Smith PhD, is the Deputy Dean of Rural and Remote Health Northern Territory, and Matthew Flinders Professor (Health and Social Equity) at Flinders University, Australia. He has worked at the research-policy-practice nexus in men's health for over two decades, with national and global expertise in men's help seeking, men's health promotion, men's health equity, and men's health policy. He was the inaugural Director of the Freemasons Centre for Male Health and Wellbeing – Northern Territory at Menzies School of Health Research, and has been an advisor to numerous national and global organisations with an interest in men's health, including the World Health Organization. In 2020, he was the NT Fulbright Senior Scholar where he visited the United States to explore health promotion strategies aimed at reducing health inequities among boys and young men of colour. In 2021, Professor Smith was presented the NT Men's Health People's Choice Award, and National Runner-Up in Men's Health Research Award, by the Australian Men's Health Forum. He is a Fellow of the Australian Health Promotion Association, Editor-in-Chief of the *Health Promotion Journal of Australia*, and Editorial Advisory Board Member of the *International Journal of Men's Social and Community Health*. He holds honorary academic status at multiple universities in Australia, Canada, and the United States.

Daphne C. Watkins PhD, is a University Diversity and Social Transformation Professor, Professor of Social Work, and Director of the Vivian A. and James L. Curtis Center for Health Equity Research and Training at the University of Michigan. Her research focuses on generating new knowledge about: (1) the social determinants of health that explain within-group differences for boys and men; (2) evidence-based strategies to improve the mental health of boys and men; and (3) the intersection of age, culture, and gender. Dr. Watkins is a mixed methods expert who uses qualitative and quantitative data to increase knowledge about how intersecting social determinants and gender dynamics place Black men at high risk for poor health. She is the past President of the American Men's Studies Association and the Founding Director of the Young Black Men, Masculinities, and Mental Health

(YBMen) Project. She also serves on several committees and boards aimed at improving men's health domestically and globally.

Derek M. Griffith PhD, is a Founder and Co-director of the Racial Justice Institute, Founder and Director of the Center for Men's Health Equity, and Professor of Health Management and Policy and Oncology at Georgetown University in Washington, D.C. Trained in psychology and public health, Dr. Griffith's program of research focuses on developing strategies to improve Black men's health and to achieve racial, ethnic, and gender equity and justice in health and well-being. Dr. Griffith is Chair of Global Action on Men's Health, and he has collaborated with colleagues in Canada, Ireland, New Zealand, and the United States on various research projects. Dr. Griffith is a contributor to and editor of *Racism: Science and Tools for the Public Health Professional* (APHA Press, 2019) and *Men's Health Equity: A Handbook* (Routledge, 2019), and author of over 150 peer-reviewed manuscripts. He has been the principal investigator of research grants from the American Cancer Society, the Robert Wood Johnson Foundation, several institutes within the National Institutes of Health, and other entities.

Contributors

Jamie M. Abelson School of Social Work, University of Michigan–Ann Arbor, Ann Arbor, MI, USA

Robbie Atatoa Pacific Health Section, School of Population Health, The University of Auckland, Auckland, New Zealand

Elizabeth S. Barnert Department of Internal Medicine & Pediatrics, David Geffen School of Medicine, University of California, Los Angeles, CA, USA

Christopher Bondoc Department of Internal Medicine & Pediatrics, David Geffen School of Medicine, University of California, Los Angeles, CA, USA

John Bosco Department of Pediatrics, David Geffen School of Medicine, University of California, Los Angeles, CA, USA

Department of Emergency Medicine, Harbour-UCLA Medical Center, Torrance, CA, USA

Brittany Ribeiro Brown School of Social Work, University of Michigan–Ann Arbor, Ann Arbor, MI, USA

Ruben Cantu Prevention Institute, Oakland, CA, USA

Frank Cohn The Dudes Club, Vancouver, BC, Canada

William Crary Prevention Institute, Oakland, CA, USA

Iloradanon H. Efimoff Department of Psychology, University of Manitoba, Winnipeg, MB, Canada

James Ellis School of Social Work, University of Michigan–Ann Arbor, Ann Arbor, MI, USA

Heriberto Escamilla National Compadres Network, San Jose, CA, USA

Teka Everstz The Dudes Club, Vancouver, BC, Canada

Jesse J. Fleay School of Education, Curtin University, Bentley, WA, Australia

Kava Fuavao Pacific Health Unit, School of Population Health, The University of Auckland, Auckland, New Zealand

Derek M. Griffith Department of Health Management and Policy, School of Health, and Center for Men's Health Equity, Racial Justice Institute, Georgetown University, Washington, DC, USA

Paul A. Gross Department of Family Practice, University of British Columbia, Vancouver, BC, Canada

The Dudes Club, Vancouver, BC, Canada

Himanshu Gupta Freemasons Centre for Male Health and Wellbeing – Northern Territory, Menzies School of Health Research, Charles Darwin University, Darwin, NT, Australia

Rural and Remote Health, College of Medicine and Public Health, Flinders University, Alice Springs, NT, Australia

Andrew Harvey School of Education, Griffith University, Logan, QLD, Australia

Braden Hill Centre of Kurongkurl Katitjin, Edith Cowan University, Mt Lawley, WA, Australia

Phyllis Shu Hubbard Radiant Health Strategies, Miramar, FL, USA

Emily C. Jaeger Center for Men's Health Equity, Racial Justice Institute, Georgetown University, Washington, DC, USA

Viviane Josewski Faculty of Medicine, University of British Columbia, Okanagan, BC, Canada

Sandy Lambert The Dudes Club, Vancouver, BC, Canada

Garrison McCleary Wilfrid Laurier University, Kitchener, Canada

Jocelyn I. Meza Department of Psychiatry, University of California, Los Angeles, CA, USA

Samuel Moore Freemasons Centre for Male Health and Wellbeing – Northern Territory, Menzies School of Health Research, Charles Darwin University, Darwin, NT, Australia

Rural and Remote Health, College of Medicine and Public Health, Flinders University, Alice Springs, NT, Australia

Vili Nosa Pacific Health Unit, School of Population Health, The University of Auckland, Auckland, New Zealand

Malakai Ofanoa Pacific Health Unit, School of Population Health, The University of Auckland, Auckland, New Zealand

John Oliffe Men's Health Research Program, School of Nursing, University of British Columbia, Vancouver, BC, Canada

Teuila Percival Pacific Health Unit, School of Population Health, The University of Auckland, Auckland, New Zealand

Lisa Puloka Pacific Health Unit, School of Population Health, The University of Auckland, Auckland, New Zealand

Peter Radoll People and Organisation, Victoria University, Melbourne, VIC, Australia

Daile L. Rung Freemason's Centre for Male Health and Wellbeing – Northern Territory, Charles Darwin University, Darwin, NT, Australia

Héctor Sánchez-Flores National Compadres Network, San Jose, CA, USA

Debra de Silva Pacific Health Unit, School of Population Health, The University of Auckland, Auckland, New Zealand

James A. Smith Rural and Remote Health, College of Medicine and Public Health, Flinders University, Darwin, NT, Australia

Menzies School of Health Research, Charles Darwin University, Darwin, NT, Australia

Freemasons Centre for Male Health and Wellbeing – Northern Territory, Menzies School of Health Research, Charles Darwin University, Darwin, NT, Australia

Garth Stahl School of Education, University of Queensland, Brisbane, QLD, Australia

Roxann McNeish Taormina Department of Child and Family Studies, College of Behavioural and Community Sciences, University of South Florida, Tampa, FL, USA

Jerry Tello National Compadres Network, San Jose, CA, USA

Bep Uink Kulbardi Aboriginal Centre, Murdoch University, Murdoch, WA, Australia

R. Bong Vergara National Compadres Network, San Jose, CA, USA

Roderick Wallace College of Education, Eastern Michigan University, Ypsilanti, MI, USA

Daphne C. Watkins School of Social Work, University of Michigan–Ann Arbor, Ann Arbor, MI, USA

Chapter 1
Introduction: What Do We Know About Global Efforts to Promote Health Among Adolescent Boys and Young Men of Colour?

James A. Smith, Daphne C. Watkins, Derek M. Griffith, and Daile L. Rung

Introduction

Research has consistently shown that men have more privilege and power than women, yet men have shorter life expectancies and higher rates of premature mortality than women in almost every country in the world (AIHW, 2017; Griffith et al., 2019; Smith et al., 2020; WHO, 2018; Department of Health, 2019). Men's adoption of risky health practices and perceived reluctance to seek help and engage in preventive health behaviours have frequently been used to explain these poorer health outcomes over the past two decades (Courtenay, 2003; Smith et al., 2008; Rovito, 2019; Vandello et al., 2019). This has been particularly notable in

J. A. Smith (✉)
Rural and Remote Health, College of Medicine and Public Health, Flinders University, Darwin, NT, Australia

Menzies School of Health Research, Charles Darwin University, Darwin, NT, Australia
e-mail: james.smith@flinders.edu.au

D. C. Watkins
School of Social Work, University of Michigan–Ann Arbor, Ann Arbor, MI, USA
e-mail: daphnew@umich.edu

D. M. Griffith
Department of Health Management and Policy, School of Health, and Center for Men's Health Equity, Racial Justice Institute, Georgetown University, Washington, DC, USA
e-mail: Derek.Griffith@georgetown.edu

D. L. Rung
Freemason's Centre for Male Health and Wellbeing – Northern Territory, Charles Darwin University, Darwin, NT, Australia
e-mail: daile.rung@cdu.edu.au

J. A. Smith et al. (eds.), *Health Promotion with Adolescent Boys and Young Men of Colour*, https://doi.org/10.1007/978-3-031-22174-3_1

discussions about adolescent boys and young adult males, whereby studies have consistently shown that they have higher rates of risky health practices such as alcohol and drug misuse, smoking, unsafe sex, reckless driving, engagement in violence, poor dietary habits, and a tendency to avoid seeking help and using health services (Cunningham & White, 2019; Rovito, 2019). Moreover, these risky health practices are disproportionately experienced among marginalised adolescent boys and young men, particularly young men of colour (Powell et al., 2010; Jones et al., 2012; Kato-Wallace et al., 2016; Cunningham & White, 2019; Gilbert et al., 2016; Rovito, 2019; Smith et al., 2021). It is essential to understand how the broader social landscape influences the risky health practices of young men of colour to ensure that they are not inaccurately apportioned blame, and to generate appropriate health intervention solutions. Scholarship on the social determinants of health clearly shows that the health and social, political, and economic inequities young men of colour face – and the subsequent health practices they adopt – are shaped by a complex array of structural factors that vary by age, race, gender, sexuality, socioeconomic status and geography (Jones et al., 2012; Kato-Wallace et al., 2016; Smith et al., 2020, 2021; Merlino et al., 2020; Smith et al., 2020).

Using examples from contemporary research and practice contexts, this book aims to unpack these complex social landscapes and structural intersections and explore what this confluence of factors means for adopting innovative and strengths-based health promotion approaches for adolescent boys and young men of colour (BYMOC). While empowerment approaches have previously been advocated when working with adolescent boys and young adult males (Armstrong & Cohall, 2011), we argue that paying greater attention to strengths-based narratives about BYMOC is a critical health promotion strategy to reduce the health inequities they often experience (Jack & Griffith, 2013; Smith et al., 2020, 2021). We purposefully bring together a range of examples from research findings and promising practices worldwide, including Australia, the United States, New Zealand, and Canada, to celebrate and highlight health promotion strategies that can help improve the life trajectories for BYMOC. In doing so, we move beyond discussing the health and social inequities faced by this population to focus on the practical actions that can be taken to address them – commonly referred to as addressing the 'know-do' gap (WHO, 2006; Bacchi, 2008; Davison et al., 2015) – and to achieve men's health equity. First, however, it is helpful to understand what we mean by addressing health and social inequities experienced by BYMOC.

Framing Health and Social Inequities in Relation to Adolescent Boys and Young Men of Colour

From the outset of this book, we acknowledge that there are multiple ways that the terms 'health equity' and 'social equity' can be defined. We also recognise that health inequities and social inequities are inextricably intertwined – that is, they often co-exist (Carey & Crammond, 2015; Carey et al., 2015; Lopez & Gadsden, 2016). For this reason, we turn to the foundational work of the WHO Commission on Social Determinants of Health to guide our thinking:

> The WHO Department of Equity, Poverty and Social Determinants of Health defines health equity as the absence of unfair and avoidable or remediable differences in health among population groups defined socially, economically, demographically, or geographically. In essence, health inequities are health differences which are: socially produced; systematic in their distribution across the population; and unfair. (Solar & Irwin, 2007, 7.)

An important concept here is that these differences – sometimes also referred to as disparities and inequalities – are regarded as health inequities if avoidable, unfair, and unjust. Health equity has long been tied to social justice, an ethical concept based on principles of distributive justice and fundamentally linked to human rights (Braveman & Gruskin, 2003).

At this juncture, it is helpful to understand the nexus between health equity and men's health. There has been a notable increase in scholarship dedicated to equity and men's health (sometimes also referred to as men's health equity) over the past decade (Williams et al., 2010; Thorpe et al., 2013; Watkins & Griffith, 2013; Baker et al., 2014; Griffith, 2016; Griffith et al., 2019; Robertson & Kilvington-Dowd, 2019; Smith et al., 2020, 2021). This work has emphasised differences between, and within, specific populations of boys and men. This scholarship is considerably different from – albeit connected with – a much broader discourse on gender equity. Indeed, policy discourses on gender equity, while important, have often perpetuated an unproductive binary between men's health and women's health, which largely fails to address the fluidity of gender relations or the poor health outcomes of men relative to women (Lohan, 2007; Broom, 2009; Smith et al., 2010; WHO, 2010; Baker et al., 2014; Smith et al., 2020). This dualistic framing has been particularly problematic for acknowledging and addressing the complex health and social inequities that marginalized men face (Smith et al., 2020). Therefore, within the context of this book, we are specifically interested in the health and social inequities experienced by adolescent BYMOC.

The health and social inequities experienced by this population are diverse and noted across various sectors. It is beyond the scope of this book to undertake a meta-analysis of such work. Indeed, this could be a book in itself. However, at a macro level, there is robust evidence to suggest that the following inequities exist among adolescent BYMOC:

- High rates of risky health practices – including those relating to:
  - Smoking (Elton-Marshall et al., 2011; Freedman et al., 2012);
  - Unsafe sex (Heerde et al., 2015; Crosby et al., 2016; Aduloju-Ajijola & Payne-Foster, 2017);
  - Alcohol and substance misuse (Chartier et al., 2011; Elton-Marshall et al., 2011); and
  - Violence (Chartier et al., 2011; Rich, 2016; Gallant et al., 2017)

- Poor mental health (Watkins et al., 2010; Prevention Institute, 2014), and high rates of suicidal ideation and suicide (Armstrong et al., 2017; Lindsey & Xiao, 2019)
- Challenges associated with health and social service access, which impinge on help-seeking practices and health service use (Hughes, 2004; Barker, 2007; Vogel et al., 2011; Canuto et al., 2018; Canuto et al., 2019; Planey et al., 2019)
- Poor education outcomes, including:

  - Low levels of participation, achievement, and completion across all levels of the education system (White, 2009; Hare & Pidgeon, 2011; Dreise & Thomson, 2014; Voisin & Elsaesser, 2014; Cook et al., n.d.; Addis & Withington, 2016; Ferguson, 2016);
  - High levels of disengagement and suspension (Fenning & Rose, 2007; Losen, 2011; Godsil, n.d.; Ferguson, 2016); and
  - Low levels of postsecondary education and career aspiration (Sikora & Biddle, 2015)

- Over-representation in the child welfare system (Tilbury, 2009), with clear evidence this impacts lifelong education, employment, and incarceration trajectories (Greenfield, 2010; Gebhard, 2013; De Vincentiis et al., 2019; Cook et al., n.d.)
- High rates of incarceration (Barker et al., 2015; De Vincentiis et al., 2019; Williams & Bergeson, 2019)
- Poor job attainment and retention, and high rates of unemployment (Bird, 2016)
- Challenges associated with accessing and retaining safe and secure housing (De Vincentiis), and homelessness (Heerde et al., 2015; De Vincentiis et al., 2019)

This information only provides a partial snapshot of some of the inequities this population faces.

In this book, our goal is not to provide a detailed summary of the different health and social inequities young men of colour face, for a variety of reasons. First, the inequities they experience are already comprehensively documented elsewhere, particularly in epidemiological and public health scholarship (see, for example, White & Holmes, 2006; AIHW, 2013; Thorpe et al., 2013; Gilbert et al., 2016; Patton et al., 2018; Cunningham & White, 2019; Ragonese et al., 2019). Second, the scholarship on racialised disparities is often specific to both context and geography. For example, there are notable differences between and among peoples of African descent and Indigenous peoples. The heterogeneity of people of African descent who have spent recent generations in the Caribbean, the United Kingdom, Canada, the United States versus the differences among Native American, Aboriginal and Torres Strait Islander, First Nations Canadian, and Maori populations are important to recognise and explicitly consider in intervention strategies. We do not want to trivialise these differences by conflating them. Instead, we intend the book to unpack, discuss and debate the synergies and tensions among them.

Third, simplistic comparisons based on sex (males vs. females) or race (White vs. colour) have led to unproductive binaries (as described above) that fail to acknowledge the complex intersections with other social and cultural dimensions. It is important to understand this multi-dimensionality to develop effective health promotion interventions for this population. Fourth, an over-emphasis on describing health and social inequities can perpetuate a deficit-based rather than a strengths-based discourse. This is at odds with the intent of this book. Instead, we want to showcase health promotion efforts that recognise and value the positive attributes tied to the range of identities of BYMOC. This means celebrating approaches that embrace concepts of empowerment, self-determination, and resilience rooted in the identities and experiences that vary by race, ethnicity, sexuality, socio-economic status, geography, and other factors. Finally, literature on gender-based health and social inequities is frequently tied to literature relating to education, employment, justice, transportation, and housing. That is, there is an array of evidence that sits outside of the health domain that can be used to inform health promotion efforts (Johnson, 2019; Richardson et al., 2019; Williams & Bergeson, 2019), particularly those seeking to promote the health and wellbeing of BYMOC (Jones et al., 2012). We deliberately capitalize on this evidence and provide practical examples that reflect this sectoral diversity throughout the chapters of this book.

We focus on research findings and novel health promotion approaches that can inform future strategies to reduce health and social inequities experienced by young men of colour (Smith et al., 2021). More specifically, we aim to convey that age (adolescent boys/young men), gender (the social construction of masculinities and manhood), and race (including cultural expressions such as Black, First Nations/Indigenous, Latino or Asian people) – and the respective intersections between them – can be intentionally and systematically incorporated to address inequities. We deliberately use intersectionality and life-course approaches as frameworks (to be explained in greater detail later in the chapter) to inform health promotion work targeting adolescent boys and young men of colour. A critical foundation of our book is the intersection of age, gender, and race, so below, we define how these terms will be used within the context of this book.

Defining Key Concepts

Age: Defining Youth

First, we acknowledge there is no universally agreed-upon definition of **youth** (Cunningham & White, 2019). However, to make this text globally applicable, we have adopted the definition of youth used by the United Nations Educational, Scientific, and Cultural Organization (UNESCO), which broadly defines youth as persons aged between 15 and 24. We use this definition to provide consistency in discussing the influence of age throughout this book. However, we also recognise that conceptualisations of youth intersect with parallel scholarship about children, adolescence, and young adulthood (Cunningham & White, 2019). Where applicable, we discuss these intersections explicitly. Indeed, the content of this book is best understood as part of a broader narrative relating to key stages of development across the life course (Braveman & Barclay, 2009; Watkins, 2012; Thorpe et al., 2015; Goodwill et al., 2018). The life-course narrative inevitably intersects with discourses on gender and race, which ultimately influences how age is viewed socially and culturally (Thorpe et al., 2015). As Thorpe, Duru, and Hill have previously argued: "a better understanding of how and why racial/ethnic disparities emerge among younger men is required to develop strategies and policy-relevant solutions that can attenuate/eliminate disparities among men of all age groups" (Thorpe et al., 2015, p. 241). As it relates to BYMOC, the concept of youth is fluid, contextual, and has lifelong consequences. As UNESCO succinctly explains (UNESCO, 2018, p. 12):

> While geography and gender characterize part of the diversity of youth, diversity also reflects the varied experiences and life situations of young people. Youth with disabilities; Indigenous youth; lesbian, gay, bisexual, and transgender youth; migrant, displaced, and refugee youth; youth in conflict and post-conflict situations; and rural youth, among others, often face challenges and barriers to participation specific to their situation. As many young people identify with more than one group, the challenges they encounter are often multiplied. The dearth of information and data on marginalized and vulnerable youth makes identifying and addressing their distinctive challenges particularly difficult.

Gender: Defining the Social and Cultural Construction of Masculinities

Within the context of this book, we define ***gender*** as the social and cultural construction of masculinities. We do this broadly, recognizing that the social construction of masculinities is a contested space, whereby adherence to hegemonic forms of masculinity (masculine norms) has frequently been used as an analytic tool in men's studies and men's health scholarship. Yet, this approach has been repeatedly challenged and is considered too simplistic to accommodate the range of gender identities adopted by boys and men (Smith et al., 2016). We are not suggesting it is an unhelpful theoretical framework – quite the contrary, understanding masculine norms in the context of individual attitudes, behaviours, and decisions in relation to health and wellbeing is important. However, we also acknowledge a burgeoning literature on multiple masculinities that offers new insights and progressive, alternative theoretical conceptualisations to more comprehensively understand patterns of health and wellbeing among young men of colour. Salient to this book are emerging yet distinct discourses relating to the social construction of manhood (Griffith, 2015; Griffith & Cornish, 2018; Vandello et al., 2019); Black masculinities (Griffith et al., 2012a; McGuire et al., 2014; Laing, 2017; Goodwill et al., 2019); and Indigenous masculinities (Innes & Anderson, 2015; Mukandi et al., 2019). Both Black and Indigenous masculinities acknowledge complex intersections between race and the social construction of gender. These emerging definitions of masculinities and manhood tend to include concepts tied to spirituality, connection to community, interdependence with their family, and the achievement of social status through their roles in community-based organisations and institutions (Gilbert et al., 2016; Griffith & Cornish, 2018; Griffith, Pennings, Bruce, & Ayers, 2019). Embracing these diverse perspectives is central to advancing global men's health promotion efforts for BYMOC (Smith et al., 2021).

Research over the past two decades has consistently shown that adherence to masculine norms is harmful to the health and wellbeing of boys and men (Ragonese et al., 2019; Heilman et al., 2019), particularly young men (Heilman et al., 2017; The Men's Project and Flood, 2018). Despite this awareness, hegemonic masculine norms have frequently been used to guide the planning and implementation of men's health promotion work (particularly as an engagement strategy), which has perpetuated masculine stereotypes known to be health-damaging to boys and men (Smith, 2007; Smith & Robertson, 2008; Fleming et al., 2014). Irrespective of whether these approaches have been intentional or inadvertent in nature, they have been heavily criticised by men's health scholars for failing to address health and social inequities experienced by marginalised groups of men (Smith, 2007; Smith & Robertson, 2008; Griffith et al., 2011; Fleming et al., 2014; Robertson & Baker, 2017). As such, research and health interventions that embrace alternative constructions of masculinities, such as Black masculinities and Indigenous masculinities, have the potential to offer novel approaches to strengths-based health promotion (Griffith et al., 2011; Smith et al., 2019a; Smith et al., 2020). We consider that embracing these alternative standpoints can help to strengthen global discourses on equity and men's health, which places a greater focus on vulnerable and marginalised groups of men, including BYMOC.

Colour: Defining Race, Ethnicity, and Culture

We use the term *colour* to represent race, culture, and ethnicity. From a socio-political perspective, this is perhaps the most contested term we have adopted throughout the book. We have used this as an umbrella term to collectively represent Black (African American), First Nations (Aboriginal and Torres Strait Islander, Maori, Native American, Native Hawaiian, Alaskan Native, and Pacific Islander), and Latinx people. While there is a consistent narrative of racial inequities and marginalisation experienced by people of colour, the socio-political and cultural underpinnings, such as slavery and colonisation, differ markedly. As such, the synergies and differences associated with race, culture, and ethnicity are openly discussed and debated throughout this book. In doing so, we demonstrate that BYMOC are as diverse as they are homogenous. Within-group and between-group heterogeneity is deliberately unpacked as part of the complex intersections between age, gender, and race. This multi-faceted focus has the greatest potential to advance health promotion efforts associated with adolescent BYMOC (Thorpe et al., 2015; Gilbert et al., 2016; Watkins et al., 2017a, b; Goodwill et al., 2018). Indeed, understanding this population in the context of key social determinants affecting their lives and wellbeing is vital (Watkins et al., 2017a, b; Watkins, 2019).

In summary, the unique characteristics and experiences of adolescent boys and young men of colour must be incorporated into developing and implementing health promotion strategies. To be effective, these health promotion approaches must be culturally-responsive, gender-specific, and age-appropriate (Griffith et al., 2012b; Goodwill et al., 2018; Watkins, 2012; Watkins et al., 2017a. We suggest that frameworks associated with intersectionality and life-course approaches are the best fit to achieve this outcome. We explain below why we have used these frameworks throughout the book.

Approaches for Advancing Equity and Men's Health Promotion

An Intersectional Approach

In line with recent global literature relating to equity and men's health, we have used an explicit intersectional lens (Griffith, 2012; Gilbert et al., 2016; Watkins et al., 2017b; Griffith et al., 2019; Robertson & Kilvington-Dowd, 2019; Smith et al., 2020). Intersectionality in men's health equity can be defined as an analytic and theoretical approach that considers the meaning and consequences of socially defined constructs – such as age, race, and gender – and offers new ways of understanding the complex causality of social phenomena (Griffith, 2012; Gilbert et al., 2016; Watkins et al., 2017b; Griffith et al., 2019). Generally speaking, intersectionality focuses on the intersecting processes that produce, reproduce and resist power, leading to the social and material disparities between groups and within them (Bauer, 2014; Robertson & Kilvington-Dowd, 2019). This focus on power relations – as they relate to intersections between age, gender, and race – is a fundamental consideration throughout this book. Noteworthy is that intersectional theoretical frameworks have been used extensively by men's health scholars (Griffith et al., 2011; Griffith, 2012; Smith et al., 2020) to unpack the health and social inequities experienced by adolescent BYMOC, including Black men (Bowleg, 2013; Bowleg et al., 2017; Griffith et al., 2013; Jennings, 2017; Watkins et al., 2017a, b), Aboriginal and Torres Strait Islander males (Smith et al., 2019a, b; Merlino et al., 2020; Smith et al., 2020), Native American men (Blume, 2019), Canadian First Nations (Smithers Graeme, 2017), Native Hawaiian and Pacific Islander men (Sinclair & Kaholokula, 2019; Sinclair & Pritchard, 2019), and Asian men (Das Nair & Thomas, 2012). Multiple scholars have argued that exploring intersections of race and gender can better guide public health work relating to men of colour, as such identities are inextricably intertwined and simultaneously dovetail with evidence on the social determinants of health (Gilbert et al., 2016, 2019).

A Life-Course Approach

Many scholars have recommended adopting a life-course approach to improve population health, particularly when aiming to achieve health equity (Braveman, 2014; Watkins, 2012; Yu, 2006). More specifically, a life-course approach has been strongly advocated as a strategy for advancing racial and ethnic minority men's health behaviours and outcomes and improved understandings of masculinities and manhood among these groups (Griffith, 2015; Thorpe et al., 2015; Gilbert et al., 2016). Thorpe et al. (2015, pp. 241–242) have convincingly argued that:

> A life-course perspective offers three key features that are important in understanding minority men's health: (1) the opportunity to identify positive or negative cumulative experiences and examine the impact of those experiences on health outcomes; (2) the timing of significant experiences in life that might contribute to patterns of health; and (3) the insight to understanding (sic) how gendered norms, beliefs, roles, and expectations evolve over-time and at different points in the life-course.

In this sense, a life-course approach offers insights into a sequence of age-linked transitions and includes times when social roles change; new rights, duties, and resources are encountered; and identities fluctuate (Settersten, 2004; Watkins, 2012). Notably, the life-course perspective focuses on understanding how early-life experiences can shape health across an entire lifetime and potentially across generations, which is particularly relevant to understanding and addressing racial disparities in health (Braveman & Barclay, 2009).

Conclusion

Globally, scholars have argued that a more critical scholarly analysis of the intersections between race, age, and gender, and other markers of difference are urgently needed to help researchers and practitioners to improve the health and wellbeing of the population and particularly BYMOC (Goodwill et al., 2018; Smith et al., 2020, 2021). This book strives to achieve this aim. It includes emerging, empirical public health-oriented research, including explorative and intervention studies using quantitative, qualitative, and mixed methods. These chapters also introduce readers to the contemporary evidence base in this field; and discuss the implications of these findings for the advancement of global health promotion research, policy, and practice contexts tailored to the needs of adolescent BYMOC. Some chapters are distinctly oriented towards health promotion practice, using examples of promising practices to showcase innovative strategies currently being adopted to reduce health and social inequities experienced by adolescent BYMOC. They deliberately draw upon diverse intersectoral examples contexts spanning health, education, employment, justice, and housing sectors to demonstrate how actions about the social and cultural determinants of health are critically important considerations to successfully engage BYMOC in health and wellbeing interventions. They also convey the importance of understanding and responding to local contextual factors and demographic characteristics when planning and implementing health promotion strategies and programs among BYMOC for this vulnerable group. Collectively, these chapters provide robust evidence-based and pragmatic strengths-based solutions for advancing health promotion efforts tailored to the needs of adolescent boys and young men of colour.

References

Addis, S., & Withington, C. (2016). *Improving high school graduation rates among males of color: Trends, findings, and recommendations*. Issues brief. Robert Wood Johnson Foundation.

Aduloju-Ajijola, N., & Payne-Foster, P. (2017). Five years later: How are we addressing the sexual health of Black boys? *Internal Medicine Review, 3*(5), 1–11.

Armstrong, B., & Cohall, A. (2011). Health promotion with adolescent and young adult males: An empowerment approach. In A. Cohall & M. Resnick (Eds.), *Advances in health promotion for adolescents and young adults – Adolescent medicine: State of the art reviews*. American Academy of Pediatrics.

Armstrong, G., Pirkis, J., Arabena, K., Currier, D., Spittal, M., & Jorm, A. (2017). Suicidal behaviour in Indigenous compared to non-Indigenous males in urban and regional Australia: Prevalence data suggest disparities increase across age groups. *Australian and New Zealand Journal of Psychiatry, 51*(12), 1240–1248.

Australian Institute of Health and Welfare (AIHW). (2013). *The health of Australia's males: From birth to young adulthood (0–24 years)*. Cat. No. PHE 168. AIHW.

Australian Institute of Health and Welfare (AIHW). (2017). *The health of Australia's males*. Australian Institute of Health and Welfare, Australian Government.

Bacchi, C. (2008). The politics of research management: Reflections on the gap between what we 'know' (about SDH) and what we do. *Health Sociology Review, 17*(2), 165–176.

Baker, P., Dworkin, S., Tong, S., Banks, I., Shand, T., & Yamey, G. (2014). The men's health gap: Men must be included in the global health equity agenda. *Bulletin of the World Health Organization, 92*, 618–620.

Barker, G. (2007). *Adolescents, social support and help-seeking behaviour: An international literature review and programme consultation with recommendations for action*. World Health Organization.

Barker, B., Alfred, G., Fleming, K., Nguyen, P., Wood, E., Kerr, T., & DeBeck, K. (2015). Aboriginal street-involved youth experience elevated risk of incarceration. *Public Health, 129*(12), 1662–1668.

Bauer, G. (2014). Incorporating intersectionality theory into population health research methodology. Challenges and the potential to advance health equity. *Social Science & Medicine, 110*, 10–17.

Bird, K. (2016). *Employment pathways for boys and young men of color: Solutions and strategies that can make a difference*. Issues brief. Robert Wood Johnson Foundation.

Blume, A. (2019). Seeking health and well-being for indigenous north American men. In D. Griffiths, M. Bruce, & R. Thorpe (Eds.), *Handbook on men's health disparities* (pp. 472–485). Routledge.

Bowleg, L. (2013). "Once you've blended the cake, you can't take the parts back to the main ingredients": Black gay and bisexual men's descriptions and experiences of intersectionality. *Sex Roles, 68*, 754–767.

Bowleg, L., del Río-González, A. M., Holt, S., Pérez, C., Massie, J., Mandell, J., & Boone, C. (2017). Intersectional epistemologies of ignorance: How behavioral and social science research shapes what we know, think we know, and don't know about U.S. Black men's sexualities. *The. Journal of Sex Research, 54*(4–5), 577–603.

Braveman, P. (2014). What is health equity: And how does a life-course approach take us further toward it? *Maternal and Child Health Journal, 18*, 366–372.

Braveman, P., & Barclay, C. (2009). Health disparities beginning in childhood: A life-course perspective. *Pediatrics, 124*(S3), S163–S175.

Braveman, P., & Gruskin, S. (2003). Defining equity in health. *Journal of Epidemiological Community Health, 57*(4), 254–258.

Broom, D. (2009). Men's health and women's health – Deadly enemies or strategic allies? *Critical Public Health, 19*(3–4), 269–278.

Canuto, K., Brown, A., Wittert, G., & Harfield, S. (2018). Understanding the utilization of primary health care services by Indigenous men: A systematic review. *BMC Public Health, 18*, 1198. https://doi.org/10.1186/s12889-018-6093-2

Canuto, K., Harfield, S., Wittert, G., & Brown, A. (2019). Listen, understand, collaborate: Developing innovative strategies to improve health service utilisation by Aboriginal and Torres Strait Islander men. *Australian and New Zealand Journal of Public Health, 43*(4), 307–309.

Carey, G., & Crammond, B. (2015). Systems change for the social determinants of health. *BMC Public Health, 15*, 662. https://doi.org/10.1186/s12889-015-1979-8

Carey, G., Crammond, B., Malbon, E., & Carey, N. (2015). Adaptive policies for reducing inequalities in the social determinants of health. *International Journal of Health Policy Management, 4*(11), 763–767.

Chartier, K., Hesselbrock, M., & Hesselbrock, V. (2011). Alcohol problems in young adults transitioning from adolescence to adulthood: The association with race and gender. *Addictive Behaviors, 36*(3), 167–174.

Cook, B., Barret, J., Hou, S., & Samson, F. (n.d.). *The intersection of the criminal justice, education, and mental healthcare systems and its influence on boys and young men of color.* Prepared for RISE for boys and men of color.

Courtenay, W. H. (2003). Key determinants of the health and wellbeing of men and boys. *International Journal of Men's Health, 2*(1), 1–30.

Crosby, R., Mena, L., Geter, A., & Hickson, D. (2016). Similarities and difference in sexual risk behaviors between young Black MSM who do and do not have sex with females. *AIDS and Behavior, 20*, 717–721.

Cunningham, M., & White, A. (2019). Young adulthood and health disparities in African American males. In D. Griffith, M. Bruce, & R. Thorpe (Eds.), *Men's health equity: A handbook* (pp. 57–71). Routledge.

Das Nair, R., & Thomas, S. (2012). Politics of desire: Exploring the ethnicity/sexuality intersectionality in south asian and east asian men who have sex with men (MSM). *Psychology of Sexualities Review, 3*(1), 8–21.

Davison, C., Ndumbe-Eyoh, S., & Clement, C. (2015). Critical examination of knowledge to action models and implications for promoting health equity. *International Journal for Equity in Health, 14*(49), 1–11.

De Vincentiis, B., Guthridge, S., Spargo, J., Su, J.-Y., & Nandakumara, S. (2019). *Story of our children and young people, Northern Territory, 2019.* Menzies School of Health Research.

Department of Health. (2019). *National men's health strategy.* Department of Health, Commonwealth of Australia.

Dreise, T., & Thomson, S. (2014). *Unfinished business: PISA shows that Indigenous youth are being left behind. Occasional essay for the Australian Council of Education Research (ACER).* ACER.

Elton-Marshall, T., Leatherdale, S., & Burkhalter, R. (2011). Tobacco, alcohol, and illicit drug use among Aboriginal youth living-off reserve: Results from the youth smoking survey. *Canadian Medical Association Journal, 183*(8), E480–E486.

Fenning, P., & Rose, J. (2007). Over-representation of African American students in exclusionary discipline: The role of school policy. *Urban Education, 42*(6), 536–559.

Ferguson, R. (2016). Aiming higher together: Strategizing better educational outcomes for boys and young men of color. : Research report prepared by Malcolm Wiener Centre for Social Policy, Harvard Kennedy School, Urban Institute.

Fleming, P., Lee, J., & Dworkin, S. (2014). "Real men don't": Constructions of masculinity and inadvertent harm in public health interventions. *American Journal of Public Health, 104*(6), 1029–1035.

Freedman, K., Nelson, N., & Feldman, L. (2012). Smoking initiation among young adults in the United States and Canada, 1998-2010: A systematic review. *Preventing Chronic Disease, 9*(110037), E05.

Gallant, D., Andrews, S., Humphreys, C., Diemer, K., Ellis, D., Burton, J., et al. (2017). Aboriginal men's programs tackling family violence: A scoping review. *Journal of Australian Indigenous Issues, 20*(2), 48–68.

Gebhard, A. (2013). Schools, prisons and Aboriginal youth: Making connections. *Journal of Educational Controversy, 7*(1), Article 4.

Gilbert, L., Ray, R., Siddiqi, A., Shetty, S., Baker, E., Elder, K., & Griffith, D. (2016). Visible and invisible trends in Black men's health: Pitfalls and promises for addressing racial, ethnic, and gender inequities in health. *Annual Review of Public Health, 37*, 295–311.

Godsil, R. (n.d.). Tools for addressing the disproportionate discipline of boys of color in schools.. Prepared for RISE for boys and men of color.

Goodwill, J. R., Watkins, D. C., Johnson, N. C., & Ober Allen, J. (2018). An exploratory study of stress and coping among Black college men. *American Journal of Orthopsychiatry, 88*(5), 538–539.

Goodwill, J., Anyiwo, N., Williams, E.-D., Johnson, N., Mattis, J., & Watkins, D. (2019). Media representations of popular culture figures and the construction of Black masculinities. *Psychology of Men & Masculinities, 20*(3), 288–298.

Greenfield, E. (2010). Child abuse as a life-course social determinant of adult health. *Maturitas, 66*(1), 51–55.

Griffith, D. (2012). An intersectional approach to men's health. *Journal of Men's Health, 9*(2), 106–112.

Griffith, D. M. (2015). "I AM a man": Manhood, minority men's health and health equity. *Ethnicity & Disease, 25*(3), 287–293.

Griffith, D. M. (2016). Biopsychosocial approaches to men's health disparities research and policy. *Behavioral Medicine, 42*(3), 211–215.

Griffith, D., & Cornish, E. (2018). "What defines a man?": Perspectives of African American men on the components and consequences of manhood. *Psychology of Men & Masculinity, 19*(1), 78–88.

Griffith, D., Metzl, J., & Gunter, K. (2011). Considering intersections of race and gender in interventions that address US men's health disparities. *Public Health, 125*(7), 417–423.

Griffith, D., Gunter, K., & Watkins, D. (2012a). Measuring masculinity in research on men of color: Findings and future directions. *American Journal of Public Health, 102*, S187–S194.

Griffith, D. M., Gunter, K., & Allen, J. O. (2012b). A systematic approach to developing contextual, culturally, and gender sensitive interventions for African American men: The example of Men 4 Health. In R. Elk & H. Landrine (Eds.), *Cancer disparities: Causes and evidence-based solutions*. Springer Publishing.

Griffith, D., Ellis, K., & Allen, J. (2013). An intersectional approach to social determinants of stress for African American men: Men's and women's perspectives. *American Journal of Men's Health, 7*(Suppl. 4), 19S–30S.

Griffith, D., Bruce, M., & Thorpe, R. (2019). Introduction. In D. Griffith, M. Bruce, & R. Thorpe (Eds.), *Men's health equity: A handbook* (pp. 3–9). Routledge.

Griffith, D., Pennings, J., Bruce, M. & Ayers, G. (2019). Measuring the dimensions of African American manhood: A factor analysis. In D. Griffith, M. Bruce, & R. Thorpe (Eds.), *Men's health equity: A handbook* (pp. 101–126). Routledge.

Hare, J., & Pidgeon, M. (2011). The way of the warrior: Indigenous youth navigating the challenges of schooling. *Canadian Journal of Education, 34*(2), 93–111.

Heerde, J., Scholes-Balog, K., & Hempill, S. (2015). Associations between youth homelessness, sexual offenses, sexual victimization, and sexual risk behaviors: A systematic literature review. *Archives of Sexual Behavior, 44*(1), 181–212.

Heilman, B., Barker, G., & Harrison, A. (2017). *The Man Box: A study on being a young man in the US, UK and Mexico*. Promundo-US and Unilever.

Heilman, B., Guerrero-Lopez, C., Ragonese, C., Kelberg, M., & Barker, G. (2019). *The cost of the Man Box: A study on the economic impacts of harmful masculine stereotypes in the United States*. Promundo-US and Unilever.

Hughes, C. (2004). Factors associated with health-seeking among Native Hawaiian men. *Pacific Health Dialog., 11*(2), 176–182.

Innes, R., & Anderson, K. (2015). *Indigenous men and masculinities: Legacies, identities, regeneration*. University of Manitoba Press.

Jack, L., & Griffith, D. (2013). The health of African American men: Implications for research and practice. *American Journal of Men's Health, 7*(Suppl. 4), 5S–7S.

Jennings, G. (2017). *An ecological and intersectionality approach to understanding African-American Men's perceptions of the intersections of gender, race, and low SES and social determinants of health*. Doctorate in Social Work (DSW) Dissertations, 90.

Johnson, W. (2019). Urban men's health: How urban environments affect Black men's health. Introduction. In D. Griffith, M. Bruce, & R. Thorpe (Eds.), *Men's health equity: A handbook* (pp. 141–179). Routledge.

Jones, D., Crump, A., & Lloyd, J. (2012). Health disparities in boys and men of color. *American Journal of Public Health, 102*(S2), S170–S172.

Kato-Wallace, J., Barker, G., Sharafi, L., Mora, L., & Lauro, G. (2016). *Adolescent boys and young men: Engaging them as supporters of gender equality and health and understanding their vulnerabilities*. Promundo-US. UNFPA.

Laing, T. (2017). Black masculinities expressed through, and restrained by, brotherhood. *The Journal of Men's Studies, 25*(2), 168–197.

Lindsey, M., & Xiao, Y. (2019). Depression, trauma, and suicide among adolescent and young adult males. In D. Griffiths, M. Bruce, & R. Thorpe (Eds.), *Men's health equity: A handbook* (pp. 288–203). Routledge.

Lohan, M. (2007). How might we understand men's health better? Integrating explanations from critical studies on men and inequalities in health. *Social Science & Medicine, 65*(3), 493–504.

Lopez, N., & Gadsden, V. (2016). *Health inequities, social determinants, and intersectionality*. Discussion Paper.

Losen, D. (2011). *Discipline policies, successful schools, and racial justice*. Colorado, National Education Policy Center.

McGuire, K., Berhanu, J., Davis, C., & Harper, S. (2014). In search of progressive Black masculinities: Critical self-reflections on gender identity development among Black undergraduate men. *Men and Masculinities, 17*(3), 253–277.

Merlino, A., Smith, J., Christie, B., Bonson, J., Adams, M., Judd, B., Aanundsen, D., Drummond, M., Osborne, R., & Fleay, J. (2020). What do we know about the nexus between culture, age, gender and health literacy? Implications for improving the health and well-being of young Indigenous males. *International Journal of Men's Social and Community Health, 3*(2) (Special Issue). https://doi.org/10.22374/ijmsch.v3i2.34

Mukandi, B., Singh, D., Brady, K., Willis, J., Sinha, T., Askew, D., & Bond, C. (2019). "So we tell them": Articulating strong Black masculinities in an urban Indigenous community. *AlterNative, 15*(3), 253–260.

Patton, G., Darmstadt, G., Petroni, S., & Dawyer, S. (2018). A gender lens on the health and well-being of young males. *Journal of Adolescent Health, 62*(3), S6–S8.

Planey, A., McNeil Smith, S., Moore, S., & Walker, T. (2019). Barriers and facilitators to mental health help-seeking among African American youth and their families: A systematic review study. *Children and Youth Services Review, 101*, 190–200.

Powell, W. H., Matthews, D., Mohottige, D., Agyemand, A., & Corbie-Smith, G. (2010). Masculinity, medical mistrust, and preventive health services delays among community-dwelling African-American men. *Journal of General Internal Medicine, 25*(12), 1300–1308.

Prevention Institute. (2014). *Making connections for mental health and wellbeing among men and boys in the US: A report on the mental health and wellbeing of men and boys in the US and opportunities to advance outcomes related to prevention, early detection and stigma reduction*. Report prepared for the Movember Foundation. Prevention Institute.

Ragonese, C., Shand, T., & Barker, G. (2019). *Masculine norms and men's health: Making the connections*. Promundo-US.

Rich, J. (2016). *Moving toward healing: Trauma and violence and boys and young men of color*. Issues brief. Robert Wood Johnson Foundation.

Richardson, N., Smith, J., Robertson, S., & Baker, P. (2019). Global men's health policy. In D. Griffiths, M. Bruce, & R. Thorpe (Eds.), *Men's health equity: A handbook* (pp. 202–222). New York.

Robertson, S., & Baker, P. (2017). Men and health promotion in the United Kingdom: 20 years further forward? *Health Education Journal, 76*(1), 102–113.

Robertson, S., & Kilvington-Dowd, L. (2019). Masculinity and men's health disparities. In D. Griffith, M. Bruce, & R. Thorpe (Eds.), *Men's health equity: A handbook* (pp. 10–26). Routledge.

Rovito, M. (2019). Male health behaviours. In D. Griffith, M. Bruce, & R. Thorpe (Eds.), *Men's health equity: A handbook* (pp. 257–274). Routledge.

Settersten, R. A. (2004). Age structuring and the rhythm of the life course. In J. T. Mortimer & M. J. Shanahan (Eds.), *Handbook of the life course* (pp. 81–98). Springer.

Sikora, J., & Biddle, N. (2015). How gendered is ambition? Educational and occupational plans for Indigenous youth in Australia. *International Journal of Educational Development, 42*, 1–3.

Sinclair, K. I. A., & Kaholokula, J. K. A. (2019). Achieving health equity for Native Hawaiian men: Aia I Hea Ka Wai A Kāne men's health equity. In D. Griffiths, M. Bruce, & R. Thorpe (Eds.), *Handbook on men's health disparities*. Routledge.

Sinclair, K., & Pritchard, D. (2019). An intersectional mixed methods approach to Native Hawaiian and Pacific Islander men's health. *Asian American Journal of Psychology, 10*(3), 268–281.

Smith, J. (2007). Beyond masculine stereotypes: Moving men's health promotion forward in Australia. *Health Promotion Journal of Australia, 18*(1), 20–25.

Smith, J., & Robertson, S. (2008). Men's health promotion: A new frontier in Australia and the UK? *Health Promotion International, 23*(3), 283–289.

Smith, J., Braunack-Mayer, A., Wittert, G., & Warin, M. (2008). "It's sort of like being a detective": Understanding how men self-monitor their health prior to seeking help and using health services. *BMC Health Services Research, 8*(56). https://doi.org/10.1186/1472-6963-8-56

Smith, J., Robertson, S., & Richardson, N. (2010). Understanding gender equity in the context of men's health policy development. *Health Promotion Journal of Australia, 21*(1), 76–77.

Smith, J., Richardson, N., & Robertson, S. (2016). Applying a gender lens to public health discourses on men's health. In J. Gideon (Ed.), *Handbook on gender and health*. Edward Elgar Publishers.

Smith, J., Christie, B., Bonson, J., Adams, M., Osborne, R., Judd, B., Drummond, M., Aanundsen, D., & Fleay, J. (2019a). *Health literacy among young Aboriginal and Torres Strait Islander males in the Northern Territory*. Menzies School of Health Research.

Smith, J., Drummond, M., Adams, M., Bonson, J., & Christie, B. (2019b). Understanding inequities in men's health in Australia: What do we know? In D. Griffith, M. Bruce, & R. Thorpe (Eds.), *Men's health equity: A handbook* (pp. 499–511). Routledge.

Smith, J. A., Watkins, D. C., & Griffith, D. M. (2020). Equity, gender, and health: New directions for global men's health promotion. *Health Promotion Journal of Australia, 31*(2), 161–165.

Smith, J., Watkins, D., & Griffith, D. (2021). Reducing health inequities facing boys and young black men in the US. *Health Promotion International, 36*(5), 1508–1515.

Smith, J., Merlino, A., Christie, B., Adams, M., Bonson, J., Osborne, R., et al. (2020). "Dudes are meant to be tough as nails": The nexus between masculinities, culture, and health literacy from the perspective of young Aboriginal and Torres Strait Islander males – Implications for policy and practice. *American Journal of Men's Health, 14(3)*, 1472–1485.

Smithers Graeme, C. (2017). *Rekindling the flame: An exploration of the relationships between health, culture and place among urban first nations men living in London, Ontario* (Electronic Thesis and Dissertation Repository). 4928.

Solar, O., & Irwin, A. (2007). *A conceptual framework for action on the social determinants of health. A discussion paper prepared for the Commission on Social Determinants of Health.* World Health Organization.

The Men's Project & Flood. (2018). *The Man Box: A study of being a young man in Australia.* Jesuit Social Services.

Thorpe, R., Richard, P., Bowie, J., Laveist, T., & Gaskin, D. (2013). Economic burden of men's health disparities in the United States. *International Journal of Men's Health, 12*(3), 195–212.

Thorpe, R., Duru, O., & Hill, C. (2015). Advancing racial/ethnic minority men's health using a life course approach. *Ethnicity & Disease, 25*(3), 241–244.

Tilbury, C. (2009). The over-representation of Indigenous children in the Australian child welfare system. *International Journal of Social Welfare, 18*(1), 57–64.

UNESCO. (2018). *World youth report: Youth and the 2030 agenda for sustainable development.* United Nations Department of Economic and Social Affairs.

Vandello, J., Bosson, J., & Lawler, J. (2019). Precarious manhood and men's health disparities. In D. Griffith, M. Bruce, & R. Thorpe (Eds.), *Men's health equity: A handbook* (pp. 27–41). Routledge.

Vogel, D. L., Heimerdinger-Edwards, S. R., Hammer, J. H., & Hubbard, A. (2011). "Boys don't cry": Examination of the links between endorsement of masculine norms, self-stigma, and help-seeking attitudes for men from diverse backgrounds. *Journal of Counseling Psychology, 58*(3), 368–382.

Voisin, D., & Elsaesser, C. (2014). Brief report: The protective effects of school engagement for African American adolescent males. *Journal of Health Psychology, 21*(4), 573–576.

Watkins, D. C. (2012). Depression over the adult life course for African American men: Toward a framework for research and practice. *American Journal of Men's Health, 6*(3), 194–210.

Watkins, D. (2019). A light on the path to and promise for Black men's mental health. *Men and Masculinities, 22*(5), 917–920.

Watkins, D. C., & Griffith, D. M. (2013). Practical solutions to addressing men's health disparities. *International Journal of Men's Health, 12*(3), 187–194.

Watkins, D., Walker, R., & Griffith, D. (2010). A meta-study of black male mental health and wellbeing. *Journal of Black Psychology., 36*(3), 303–330.

Watkins, D., Allen, J., Goodwill, J., & Noel, B. (2017a). Strengths and weaknesses of the Young Black Men, Masculinities, and Mental Health (YBMen) Facebook project. *American Journal of Orthopsychiatry, 87*(4), 392–401.

Watkins, D. C., Mitchell, J. A., Hawkins, J., & Mouzon, D. M. (2017b). *A field scan of physical and mental health interventions for adult Black men in the United States. Commissioned report submitted to RISE for boys and men of color.* University of Pennsylvania.

White, H. (2009). *Increasing the achievement of African American males* (Research brief No. 3). Report from the Department of Research.

White, A., & Holmes, M. (2006). Patterns of mortality across 44 countries among men and women aged 15-44 years. *Journal of Men's Health & Gender, 3*(2), 139–151.

Williams, J., & Bergeson, C. (2019). Incarceration as determinant of poor health outcomes. Introduction. In D. Griffith, M. Bruce, & R. Thorpe (Eds.), *Men's health equity: A handbook* (pp. 180–188). Routledge.

Williams, R., Robertson, S., & Hewison, A. (2010). Men's health, inequalities and policies: Contradictions, masculinities and public health in England. *Critical Public Health, 19*(3–4), 475–488.

World Health Organization (WHO). (2006). *Bridging the "know-do" gap: Meeting on knowledge translation in global health.* WHO Document Production Services.

World Health Organization (WHO). (2010). *Policy approaches to engaging men and boys in achieving gender equality and health equity.* World Health Organization.

World Health Organization (WHO). (2018). *The health and wellbeing of men in the WHO European region: Better health through a gender approach.* WHO Regional Office for Europe.

Yu, S. (2006). The life-course approach to health. *American Journal of Public Health, 96*(5), 768.

Chapter 2
Becoming: An Intervention to Promote Mental Wellbeing of Young Black Men in the United States

Derek M. Griffith and Emily C. Jaeger

Introduction

On August 23, 2020, Jacob Blake, a 29-year-old Black father, was shot seven times by a White police officer in front of three of his children outside of an apartment complex in Kenosha, Wisconsin (Morales, 2021). The year prior, several Black men – including Elijah McClain, Ahmaud Arbery, and George Floyd – were shot at the hands of White vigilantes or police officers. In the days following Jacob Blake's shooting, video of the event circulated widely on social media and professional athletes – particularly young Black men – in professional basketball and professional baseball led protests and spoke out. Twenty-five-year-old Dominic Smith, a player for the New York Mets, said, "I think the most difficult part is to see people still don't care. For this to just continuously happen, it just shows the hate in people's hearts. That just sucks, you know? Being a Black man in America, it's not easy" (Sherman, 2020).

For Black men in the United States, this is not a new phenomenon (Young, 2017). Characterisations of Black men as violent, delinquent, or troublemakers historically have been used to vindicate the use of deadly force against them, even when unarmed, as in the case of George Floyd and others (Gilbert & Ray, 2016; Hartfield et al., 2018; Krieger, 2020). Regardless of individual or collective efforts to demonstrate the contrary, the American public has viewed Black men as "threatening,

This chapter has been supported in part by the Center for Men's Health Equity at Georgetown University and the Movember Foundation.

D. M. Griffith (✉) · E. C. Jaeger
Center for Men's Health Equity, Racial Justice Institute, Georgetown University, Washington, DC, USA
e-mail: Derek.Griffith@georgetown.edu; ej302@georgetown.edu

17

J. A. Smith et al. (eds.), *Health Promotion with Adolescent Boys and Young Men of Colour*, https://doi.org/10.1007/978-3-031-22174-3_2

hostile, aggressive, unconscientious and incorrigible" (Young, 2017, p. 42); in other words, lacking character. In this context, character assassination is "an act of consistently presenting false or indicting arguments about a person in order to encourage his or her public dislike or distrust" (Young, 2017, p. 42). Regardless of whether Black men conduct themselves in a respectful and socially appropriate manner, Black men have to manage the negative stereotypes that others have of them (Jackson & Harvey Wingfield, 2013).

Since March 2020, COVID-19 has taken over the lives of people globally. From the earliest articles documenting mortality from the virus, data on COVID-19 have found that men have been dying from the virus at higher rates than women (Griffith et al., 2020; Morgan et al., 2021; Smith et al., 2020a). In June 2020, men reported slightly lower rates of anxiety than women, but had higher rates of depressive symptoms (Czeisler et al., 2020) and suicidal ideation (Czeisler et al., 2020). Symptoms of depression in men tend to include aggression, engaging in high-risk activities, and utilisation of alcohol or drugs (Martin et al., 2013; National Institute of Mental Health, 2017). Often, men's presentation of depressive symptoms is consistent with clinical reports, yet they may not be included in traditional diagnostic screeners or criteria (Martin et al., 2013). Black/African Americans reported the greatest increase in anxiety and depression, and young people, military veterans, trauma survivors, and GBTQIA+ males have reported particularly high rates of suicidal ideation (Mental Health America, 2021). According to Mental Health America (Mental Health America, 2021), the rates of reporting frequent thoughts of suicide are the highest they have recorded in their seven-year history. Women are three to four times more likely to attempt suicide than men, but because men often choose more lethal means to attempt suicide, the suicide mortality rate of men is nearly four times the rate of women (Callanan & Davis, 2012). In this context, it remains crucial to better understand how to promote the mental health and wellbeing of young Black men (Goodwill et al., 2021; Smith et al., 2020b).

Interventions to promote mental health and wellbeing have often focused on changing gendered ideals and norms as well as identifying and managing symptoms of poor mental health. While it is important to address these downstream factors, what appears to be missing from these interventions is the appreciation of the structural context of young Black men's lives. Their context is not shaped solely by their maleness or manhood, however precarious, but also by structural racism. In this chapter, we outline and argue for a structural intervention that adapts to the context of young Black men's lives, and which considers how the structural racism they experience is uniquely gendered and anti-Black (Griffith et al., 2021). Beginning with defining mental health, wellbeing and self-care, and framing the biopsychosocial context of young men's development, we discuss key aspects of anti-Black gendered structural racism for young Black men. Then, we outline *Becoming*, a structural intervention to promote wellbeing among 18-to-25-year-old Black men in the United States.

Background and Literature Review

Mental Health and Wellbeing

Mental health is more than just the absence of mental disorders or disabilities. According to the World Health Organization (WHO), mental health is a state of well-being in which an individual realizes their own abilities, can cope with the normal stresses of life, can work productively, and is able to contribute to their communities (World Health Organization, 1946, 1986).

Mental health includes our emotional, psychological, and social well-being. Despite its importance, health (whether mental health or physical health) is not the object of living or a goal in and of itself. Health/mental health is a resource for everyday life (World Health Organization, 1986) that is important because it allows people to pursue life goals and wellbeing. "Wellbeing is about the reasons one wishes to be alive" (Kottke et al., 2016), and includes subjective, personal (self-reported aspects of life satisfaction) and objective (health, income, safety, housing) components (Robert Wood Johnson Foundation, 2019). Personal or individual wellbeing can be defined as including how satisfied we are with our lives, our sense that what we do in life is worthwhile, individual perception of meaning and purpose in our lives, our day-to-day emotional experiences (happiness and anxiety), and an overall sense of mental health (i.e., subjective wellbeing like self-rated health) (Everett, 2015). Psychological wellbeing is not solely the absence of depression, anxiety and other symptoms or diagnoses, but the presence of meaning, happiness, belonging, and other positive psychological states (Arslan, 2021). It also helps determine how we handle stress, relate to others, and make choices. Peak mental health is not about avoiding stressors or challenges, but it is about looking after ongoing wellness and happiness.

Health and wellbeing can be defined as how individuals think (e.g., autonomy, self-worth, experience optimism), feel (i.e., sense of security and satisfaction with life) and function (i.e., physiological conditions and ability to meet personal and collective needs) – both personally and socially – and how they evaluate their lives as a whole (National Academies of Sciences, Engineering & Medicine, 2020). Individuals consider numerous aspects of health when they judge their overall health; this judgment seems to be more consistent with definitions of health that also consider wellbeing than those that have a narrower conceptualisation of health.

Thriving corresponds to psychological wellbeing and is defined as functioning in the fullest state of mental, physical and social wellbeing (Arslan, 2021). Consequently, thriving is often conceptualized as the outcome of positive interventions that aim to cultivate positive thoughts, feelings, practices, and behaviours that have been demonstrated to increase wellbeing (Heekerens & Heinitz, 2019). Thriving includes autonomy, or the belief that one has control over their life (Arslan, 2021; Ryan & Deci, 2000). Seligman (2011) proposed five pillars of wellbeing represented by the acronym PERMA: positive emotions, engagement, positive relationships, meaning in life, and accomplishments. Consequently, one key aspect of thriving is engaging in self-care: regular practices that become part of everyday life that are consciously and intentionally done to impact wellbeing.

Biopsychosocial Aspects of Young Men's Lives

Generally, young adults tend to be less healthy than adolescents (Cunningham & White, 2019). The early 20s is a developmental period during which genetically-based mental health issues begin to present. Those with a family history of mental illness may begin to exhibit symptoms reflective of mental health challenges. Moreover, the brain is not fully developed until the early 20s in males. In particular, the frontal lobe – the area of the brain associated with reasoning – is not complete until this age (Cunningham & White, 2019). Because the amygdala (the part of the brain that controls emotions) develops before the frontal lobe (the part of the brain that controls reasoning), decision-making may be associated with what feels good, rather than what is appropriate and right (Cunningham & White, 2019). This unevenness in brain development has been offered as a possible explanation for risk-taking behaviours during young adulthood, which may also be an example of exploration of masculine beliefs and attitudes (Cunningham & White, 2019).

From a psychological and social development standpoint, the primary psychosocial developmental goal of people in this age group is to transition from childhood and adolescence to being an adult. Becoming an adult, becoming a man (an adult male), is a process, not a discrete event (Settersten et al., 2015). Being an adult also is something that is defined by oneself and others. Because 18–25 are the ages that mark the early stages of being an adult, some have described early adulthood as a "novice phase" in which the primary task is to move beyond adolescence and build a stable life structure (Levinson, 1986). A stable life structure is one where people in this age group are expected to become financially independent, establish romantic relationships, become parents, and assume responsible roles as productive and engaged members of the community (Bonnie et al., 2014). As part of this process of transitioning to adult roles and responsibilities, young adults experience the weakening of the safety net that has supported them throughout their lives to date (Cunningham & White, 2019).

Along with these expectations, some of the markers of adulthood are associated with more abstract concepts like *maturity, independence, responsibility, and personal control* (Settersten et al., 2015). In these ways, young people use more individualistic criteria for defining adulthood and framing their sense of adulthood than more traditional roles may suggest (Settersten et al., 2015). While independence is often touted as the marker of adulthood, the reality is quite different. Adulthood is perhaps better characterized as interdependence – where you can rely on others and others can rely on you (Settersten et al., 2015). Relationships with family, friends, and others affect who we are and what we become; these social networks open and constrain choices and opportunities (Settersten et al., 2015). It is critical to help young Black men recognize the value of social supports and networks in key aspects of their personal and professional lives.

The characteristics of a particular nation, state, and locale, and a particular time in history shape expectations. It is noteworthy that the current generation of young adults have tended to delay pursuing key adult roles and responsibilities (e.g., marriage, home ownership, beginning careers). In recent years, young adults also have faced considerable student loan debt, stagnant wages, increased social isolation, and sedentary behaviour associated with technology use (e.g., social media, video games, binge watching shows/movies) (Dimock, 2019). Dependency on smartphones for internet use is common among young adults, lower-income African Americans and African American men (Pew Research Center, 2016).

In addition, many people do not see or treat 18-to-25-year-olds as adults, in part because their lives do not match traditional views of adulthood (i.e., being financially independent and being responsible for others) (National Research Council, 2015; Stroud et al., 2015). Similarly, many, if not most, 18-to-25-year-olds today do not completely feel like adults. They may feel like adults at work, with romantic partners, or with children, but they may not feel like adults when interacting with parents or friends (Settersten et al., 2015). The completion of school or training is another social marker of adulthood (Settersten et al., 2015) and with so many young adults in school or training, it is often difficult to measure socio-economic status (SES) in this age group (Cunningham & White, 2019). Yet, financial needs and expectations may cause tension and stress for young men and in their families. These financial stressors, and the psychological and social meaning associated with them, can be important sources of stress, strain, and burnout.

Black men may cope with chronically stressful economic and social conditions at the expense of their personal health (Griffith et al., 2011). This should not be interpreted as Black men not believing that health and wellbeing are important; rather this suggests that Black men see fulfilling these roles as more important to their families and communities than prioritising success in fulfilling key gendered social roles. Manhood's historical ties to economic success, material wealth and social class status (Summers, 2013; Summers, 2004) have remained consistent across generations. For young Black men, there are three different types of strains they may potentially experience: student role strain (prioritising schooling and educational preparation over wellbeing), worker role strain (prioritising looking for, securing, and maintaining adequately paying employment over well-being), and provider role strain (prioritising contributing financially to a household and taking care of responsibilities for children and family over wellbeing) (Griffith et al., 2011; Watkins, 2012). This is consistent with the notion of John Henryism and the fable of John Henry, which is explained further below (Griffith et al., 2012; James et al., 1983).

Black men often find through their lives and experiences that the promise that the United States is a meritocracy is a myth (Kwate & Meyer, 2010); hard work is not equally beneficial to everyone (Cawthorne, 2009; Isaacs et al., 2007; Williams, 2003). Being too focused on achieving goals and professional success can have physical and mental health costs. Some have characterized this as John Henryism

(Singer et al., 2020). The concept of John Henryism is the idea that someone would seek to overcome a chronic stressor or barrier in life by simply working harder and longer, and perhaps spending less time and energy thinking through alternative strategies or resources that might be marshalled to help complete the task (James, 1994). While John Henry demonstrated positive characteristics of manhood and demonstrated his work ethic, he also demonstrated how he prioritised his career above his health, highlighting the obvious paradox: in trying to demonstrate positive values his health suffered. Self-reliance is certainly a pillar of how young men are taught to view key gendered ideals and to demonstrate an ability to be successful with as little help as possible.

While some have characterized this psychological trait as John Henryism, others have characterized this as burnout when it occurs in work contexts (Awa et al., 2010). Given that burnout is a combination of emotional exhaustion (depleted emotional resources), depersonalisation (negative, cynical and detached approach to others), and reduced personal accomplishment (a low sense of confidence in oneself and negative feelings about oneself) (Awa et al., 2010). An imbalance between job demands and job skills, lack of control over tasks at work, lack of reward/ acknowledgement of effort, and prolonged work stress are some of the leading factors leading to burnout (Awa et al., 2010). While it remains a contested concept, burnout has been recognized by WHO and others as a determinant of mental wellbeing specific to the occupational context (Heinemann & Heinemann, 2017; World Health Organization, 2019). Burnout is not considered a medical condition (Heinemann & Heinemann, 2017), but it is considered a determinant of health that influences health status or contact with health services (World Health Organization, 2019).

Anti-Black Gendered Structural Racism and Health

Racism produces social conditions that predispose Black people to disability and death from COVID-19 and other health and social factors (Poteat et al., 2020), and reflects the totality of ways that ideologies of inherent racial inferiority of social groups called races are ranked and differentially allocated societal resources through mutually reinforcing sectors of society (e.g., health care, housing, education, criminal justice) in ways that determine population-level patterns of health and wellbeing (Bailey et al., 2017; Griffith, 2021; Williams & Rucker, 2000). Racism is a fundamental part of the macrosocial context of the experience of people of African descent in the United States (Hutchinson, 1997; Pieterse & Carter, 2007). Racism adversely affects the health and wellbeing of Black men and others through negative beliefs and stereotypes that are rooted in U.S. culture (Williams & Cooper, 2020). When compared with men of other racial and ethnic groups and when compared with Black women, Black men may experience more intense discrimination because their social interactions tend to be based on a range of negative race- and gender-based stereotypes that characterise Black men as having fundamental constitutional weaknesses that make them prone to hostility, criminality, violence, and other antisocial behaviours (Griffith & Johnson, 2013; Pieterse & Carter, 2007; Young, 2017). Some research has shown that Black men experience more daily indignities and microaggressions than Black women (Weitzer & Brunson, 2015). In the United States, Black men are more likely than any other group to be targeted, profiled, incriminated, investigated, unjustly committed, harshly sentenced, and imprisoned for crimes (Carson, 2014; Miller & Vittrup, 2020). Because Black men have historically been viewed as violent and delinquent or stereotyped as uncooperative troublemakers, it appears to vindicate the use of deadly force on them (Gilbert & Ray, 2016; Hartfield et al., 2018). In qualitative research by Watkins and Neighbors (2007), young Black men discussed that their notions of depression were tied to societal images of Black men and the lack of support they feel from their networks to combat depressive symptoms. They also did not want to show weakness, vulnerability, or pain because "society" may use those as weapons against them (Goodwill et al., 2018; Watkins et al., 2010).

One way that racism affects health is through stress mechanisms (Bailey et al., 2017; Harrell, 2000; Kirkinis et al., 2018). Stress process models highlight how stressors relate to identity, meaning they involve damages or losses to highly valued identities (McLeod, 2012). Chronic stress can cause excess wear and tear on body organs and systems, leading to hypertension, obesity, diabetes, and other adverse health outcomes (Alang et al., 2017; Duru et al., 2012). Racism-related stress has been associated with health-related outcomes and physiological wellbeing such as hypertension (Hicken et al., 2019), depressive symptoms (Wheaton et al., 2018), cigarette smoking (Parker et al., 2017), and alcohol use (Pittman et al., 2019). Experiencing or witnessing police brutality in person or through the media, hearing stories of friends who have experienced brutality, and having to worry about becoming a victim are all stressors (Alang et al., 2017). Given the racial disparities in COVID-19 mortality, the federal response to the pandemic may be viewed as a form of systemic racism and its own source of stress for Black men (Ruxton & Burrell, 2020).

Becoming

It is critical that interventions to promote young Black men's mental health and wellbeing consider the structural context that shapes their daily lives and life chances (Goodwill et al., 2018). The three health behaviours we seek to promote in *Becoming* are self-care, offering support to others, and seeking help from trusted others. Self-care is an umbrella term for any conscious, intentional, and regular behaviour that young Black men may engage in to help them live well and to improve their mental and physical health (National Institute of Mental Health, 2021). Some behaviours that we would encourage and promote are regular exercise, healthy eating practices, adequate sleep, meditation, goal-setting, being grateful, staying positive, and remaining connected to family and friends (National Institute of Mental Health, 2021). These behaviours help young Black men create lifestyles that give them the best chances to prevent mental health problems from adversely affecting their daily functioning, and to have the social supports to manage them or determine if they need professional help. It is critical for young Black men to develop strong social support networks and maintain existing relationships and networks by staying connected with others and spending time with people who make them feel positive; talking with people they trust when times get tough (although we must first help them to identify people they trust); and helping support others when times get tough. While young Black men need help identifying sources of support, they also need to be able to identify sources of stress and discouragement (Bowman, 1989). Some of those sources of stress and discouragement may be from historical trauma (Barlow, 2018), experiences of discrimination, the absence of positive messages and images, or the absence of people who are encouraging and believe in the young men and their vision (Watkins et al., 2020).

The process of *Becoming* also combines Akbar's three step process of critical self-education – deconstructionist, reconstructionist, and constructionist (Akbar, 1998) – with Watts's research on socio-political development (Griffith & Semlow, 2020; Watts et al., 1999; Watts et al., 2003). Socio-political development is a process of increasing knowledge, analytic skills, emotional faculties, and capacity to engage in behaviours that directly or indirectly seek to achieve change in social and political systems (Watts et al., 2003) that lead to health equity. The goal of *Becoming* is to facilitate critical thought that leads to action (Watts & Hipolito-Delgado, 2015).

Deconstructionist Phase

The *deconstructionist* phase is characterized by critical social analysis: helping people to critically analyse and challenge their social world; not adapt to it (Freire, 1970; Watts et al., 1999, 2003). A key part of this analysis is understanding that the root causes of social and health inequities flow from a system of inequality that unfairly disadvantages some and unfairly advantages others (Watts & Hipolito-Delgado, 2015). This is particularly important in combatting some of the individual and collective processes associated with John Henryism (James, 1994). One of the flawed assumptions associated with John Henryism is the assumption that the solution to life stressors and challenges are solved via personal responsibility, tenacity, and behaviours associated with an internal locus of control (Neighbors et al., 1996). Racism, however, is a structure of inequality that cannot be dismantled or overcome simply by individual behaviour because the root cause of the problem is structural, not individual. While some may argue that recognizing the structural inequities that comprise a system of racism justifies a lack of effort or character, there is little evidence to support this assumption. Rather, a fatalistic attitude that recognizes the structural limitations is both healthy and adaptive, even if the goal is to either adapt to or dismantle the system (Came & Griffith, 2017; Neighbors et al., 1996; Watts et al., 1999). Helping young Black men see how racism is part of the fabric of our society is essential to dismantling it and eliminating its effects on health. Accurately defining the scope and nature of a problem is a key foundation for creating an effective solution.

Reconstructionist Phase

Once people have developed critical awareness of these issues, the *reconstructionist* phase helps young men propose strategies to address the limitations and errors they identified. This phase is rooted in the notion of critical resilience (Antabe et al., 2021). While some have psychologised (Mills, 2000) the notion of resilience and not considered the structural context of this call for agency, Antabe et al. (2021) root their conception of resilience in efforts of Black populations to recognize, mitigate, resist, and undo the structural conditions that adversely affect their health and wellbeing. From this perspective, resilience is based on the assets and resources of individuals and communities that facilitate their ability to understand their circumstances and to meaningfully identify, respond to, and challenge the social arrangements, social norms, and ideologies that compromise their wellbeing (Antabe et al., 2021). Antabe et al. (2021) argue that resistance is not limited to merely identifying or expressing opposition to structural racism, but it also includes imagining alternative futures and possibilities for creating a just society where all have equal opportunities to be healthy and well.

Fundamental to *Becoming* is the idea that young Black men need to connect with others. Thus, listening, building human relationships, nurturing trust, respect and understanding (Came & Griffith, 2017) are essential components of the process. Encouraging active sharing and participation of all involved and the presumption that all have some level of expertise to bring to the ultimate goals are keys to this phase. Horizontal communication, rather than privileging some voices over others, also may be critical to model and encourage if the goal is to work across the heterogeneity of young Black men to create common strategies and goals (Watts & Hipolito-Delgado, 2015).

One of the key goals of this phase is collective identification, or facilitating feelings of solidarity, collective efficacy and shared culture (Watts & Hipolito-Delgado, 2015) while simultaneously celebrating individuality. Some of the components of collective efficacy include an increase in positive regard for one's social group and their membership in it, and embracing the goal of inspiring change, not simply for oneself, but for the betterment of the group (Watts & Hipolito-Delgado, 2015). It is critical to help young men envision and sympathise with the harsh realities of disadvantaged individuals and situations, and to enhance emotional identification with and build empathy and support for populations that experience disproportionately poor health outcomes. And yet, it is equally important to recognise that their shared experience is not only one of oppression, but one of resistance, resilience, and strength.

Constructionist Phase

The final phase of *Becoming* is the *constructionist* phase. The goal of this phase is praxis, or the creation of ways of thinking for the purpose of action, and the expectation that insights from action will help to refine how we think about the problem and potential solutions (Watts & Hipolito-Delgado, 2015). Social capital is a key component of this effort to synthesise knowledge and begin individual and collective action to promote wellbeing. Social capital refers to the potentially positive aspects of social life that are derived from shared social networks, social norms, and trust (Bamford et al., 2021). Social capital is often described as including both cognitive social capital (aspects of trust, trustworthiness, social support neighbourhood support etc.) and structural social capital (connection with, membership in, and attendance in churches or social organisations) (Bamford et al., 2021). While structural social capital is important, cognitive social capital has been documented to be an important predictor of mental wellbeing, and high levels of social capital may enhance a sense of belonging and thus increase collective wellbeing (Bamford et al., 2021).

For people to be motivated to get involved – and remain involved – in efforts to create change and help to mobilise others, they must first feel motivated to respond (Kieffer, 1984). Often that comes from the desire to "become free not simply *from* something, but *for* something" (p. 166) (italics in original) (Harding, 1990). Thus, it is critical to promote political efficacy, or an increased confidence and motivation to act to pursue health equity (Watts & Hipolito-Delgado, 2015). Feeling capable of action – and that the action will be meaningful and impactful – are essential precursors to action, but these also require hope and optimism (Christens et al., 2013). Hope and optimism are hard to create and often harder to sustain (Christens et al., 2013), but nonetheless are essential to promoting wellbeing.

Conclusion

In her book *On Becoming*, Michele Obama argues that becoming is not about the destination, but it is about a continual process towards a better self (Obama, 2021). In other words, becoming is a commitment to the lifelong process where one begins to be, grows to be, turns into, or comes to be (Obama, 2021). Because this is a lifelong process, the principle of *Becoming* is to help young Black men change their behaviour or develop new behaviours in the short-term, and to learn information, identify sources of motivation, and develop the skills and supports to make lifelong lifestyle changes. This notion is useful for promoting health efforts among young Black men because it provides a touchstone or foundation that they can return to as new situations and challenges arise. As young Black men navigate life and become men, becoming can be a cornerstone that helps them build from positive resources, assets, and strengths in themselves and in their interpersonal relationships. Thus, the principle of becoming can help young Black men understand the critical importance of staying connected to positive, supportive, like-minded people. In these relationships, it is critical that they both offer support to others and seek help from them, too. These insights, relationships, and behaviours must acknowledge the structural limitations that constrain them, and yet foster the hope, courage, and optimism to move forward.

References

Akbar, N. (1998). *Man know thyself*. Mind Productions.

Alang, S., McAlpine, D., McCreedy, E., & Hardeman, R. (2017). Police brutality and black health: Setting the agenda for public health scholars. *American Journal of Public Health, 107*(5), 662–665.

Antabe, R., Miller, D., Kohoun, B., Okonufua, O., & Husbands, W. (2021). Black resilience: A strategic asset for engaging heterosexual Black Canadian men in community responses to HIV. *Journal of Racial and Ethnic Health Disparities., 9*, 756–766. https://doi.org/10.1007/s40615-021-01011-w

Arslan, G. (2021). Psychological well-being in college students: Psychometric properties of the Brief Inventory of Thriving (BIT) and the Comprehensive Inventory of Thriving (CIT). *Journal of School and Educational Psychology, 1*(1), 6–16. https://doi.org/10.47602/josep.v1i1.6

Awa, W. L., Plaumann, M., & Walter, U. (2010). Burnout prevention: A review of intervention programs. *Patient Education and Counseling, 78*(2), 184–190.

Bailey, Z. D., Krieger, N., Agénor, M., Graves, J., Linos, N., & Bassett, M. T. (2017). Structural racism and health inequities in the USA: Evidence and interventions. *The Lancet, 389*(10077), 1453–1463. https://doi.org/10.1016/S0140-6736(17)30569-X

Bamford, J., Klabbers, G., Curran, E., Rosato, M., & Leavey, G. (2021). Social capital and mental health among Black and minority ethnic groups in the U.K. *Journal of Immigrant and Minority Health, 23*(3), 502–510. https://doi.org/10.1007/s10903-020-01043-0

Barlow, J. N. (2018). Restoring optimal black mental health and reversing intergenerational trauma in an era of Black Lives Matter. *Biography, 41*(4), 895–908.

Bonnie, R. J., Stroud, C. E., & Breiner, H. E. (2014). *Investing in the health and well-being of young adults*. National Academies Press.

Bowman, P. J. (1989). Research perspectives on Black men: Role strain and adaptation across the adult life cycle. In R. L. Jones (Ed.), *Black adult development and aging* (pp. 117–150). Cobb & Henry Publishers.

Brandon A., Jackson Adia, Harvey Wingfield (2013) Getting Angry to Get Ahead: Black College Men Emotional Performance and Encouraging Respectable *Masculinity. Symbolic Interaction 36*(3) 275–292. https://doi.org/10.1002/symb.63

Callanan, V. J., & Davis, M. S. (2012). Gender differences in suicide methods. *Social Psychiatry and Psychiatric Epidemiology, 47*(6), 857–869.

Came, H., & Griffith, D. (2017). Tackling racism as a "wicked" public health problem: Enabling allies in anti-racism praxis. *Social Science & Medicine, 199*, 181–188. https://www.sciencedirect.com/science/article/abs/pii/S0277953617301740?via%3Dihub

Carson, E. A. (2014). *Prisoners in 2013 (NCJ 247282)*. U.S. Department of Justice.

Cawthorne, A. (2009). *Weathering the storm: Black men in the recession*. Center for American Progress.

Christens, B. D., Collura, J. J., & Tahir, F. (2013). Critical hopefulness: A person-centered analysis of the intersection of cognitive and emotional empowerment. *American Journal of Community Psychology, 52*(1–2), 170–184.

Cunningham, M., & White, A. (2019). Young adulthood and health disparities in African American males. In D. Griffith, M. Bruce, & R. Thorpe (Eds.), *Men's health equity: A handbook* (pp. 57–71). Routledge.

Czeisler, M. É., Lane, R. I., Petrosky, E., Wiley, J. F., Christensen, A., Njai, R., Weaver, M. D., Robbins, R., Facer-Childs, E. R., & Barger, L. K. (2020). Mental health, substance use, and suicidal ideation during the COVID-19 pandemic—United States, June 24–30, 2020. *Morbidity and Mortality Weekly Report, 69*(32), 1049.

Dimock, M. (2019). Defining generations: Where millennials end and generation Z begins. *Pew Research Center, 17*(1), 1–7.

Duru, O. K., Harawa, N. T., Kermah, D., & Norris, K. C. (2012). Allostatic load burden and racial disparities in mortality. *Journal of the National Medical Association, 104*(1–2), 89–95.

Everett, G. (2015). Measuring national well-being: A U.K. perspective. *Review of Income and Wealth, 61*(1), 34–42.

Freire, P. (1970). *Pedagogy of the oppressed.* Herder and Herder.

Gilbert, K. L., & Ray, R. (2016). Why police kill black males with impunity: Applying Public Health Critical Race Praxis (PHCRP) to address the determinants of policing behaviors and "justifiable" homicides in the USA. *Journal of Urban Health, 93*(1), 122–140.

Goodwill, J. R., Watkins, D. C., Johnson, N. C., & Allen, J. O. (2018). An exploratory study of stress and coping among Black college men. *American Journal of Orthopsychiatry, 88*(5), 538–549. https://doi.org/10.1037/ort0000313

Goodwill, J. R., Taylor, R. J., & Watkins, D. C. (2021). Everyday discrimination, depressive symptoms, and suicide ideation among African American men. *Archives of Suicide Research, 25*(1), 74–93. https://doi.org/10.1080/13811118.2019.1660287

Griffith, D. M. (2021). Well-being in healthy people 2030: A missed opportunity. *Health Education & Behavior, 48*(2), 115–117. https://doi.org/10.1177/1090198121997744

Griffith, D. M., & Johnson, J. L. (2013). Implications of racism for African American men's cancer risk, morbidity and mortality. In H. M. Treadwell, C. Xanthos, K. B. Holden, & R. L. Braithwaite (Eds.), *Social determinants of health among African American men (pp. 21–38).* Jossey-Bass.

Griffith, D. M., & Semlow, A. R. (2020). Art, anti-racism and health equity: "Don't ask me why, ask me how!". *Ethnicity & Disease, 30*(3), 373–380. https://doi.org/10.18865/ed.30.3.373

Griffith, D. M., Gunter, K., & Allen, J. O. (2011). Male gender role strain as a barrier to African American men's physical activity. *Health Education & Behavior, 38*(5), 482–491. https://doi.org/10.1177/1090198110383660

Griffith, D. M., Gunter, K., & Watkins, D. C. (2012). Measuring masculinity in research on men of color: Findings and future directions. *American Journal of Public Health, 102*(Suppl. 2), S187–S194. https://doi.org/10.2105/AJPH.2012.300715

Griffith, D. M., Sharma, G., Holliday, C. S., Enyia, O. K., Valliere, M., Semlow, A. R., Stewart, E. C., & Blumenthal, R. S. (2020). Men and COVID-19: A biopsychosocial approach to understanding sex differences in mortality and recommendations for practice and policy interventions. *Preventing Chronic Disease, 17*, E63.

Griffith, D. M., Holliday, C. S., Enyia, O. K., Ellison, J. M., & Jaeger, E. C. (2021). Using syndemics and intersectionality to explain the disproportionate COVID-19 mortality among Black men. *Public Health Reports, 136*(5), 523–531. https://doi.org/10.1177/00333549211026799

Harding, V. (1990). *History and hope: Why we must share the story of the movement.* Orbis Books.

Harrell, S. P. (2000). A multidimensional conceptualization of racism-related stress: Implications for the well-being of people of color. *American Journal of Orthopsychiatry, 70*(1), 42–57.

Hartfield, J. A., Griffith, D. M., & Bruce, M. A. (2018). Gendered racism is a key to explaining and addressing police-involved shootings of unarmed Black men in America. In *Inequality, crime, and health among African American males* (Research in race and ethnic relations) (Vol. 20, pp. 155–170). Emerald Publishing Limited.

Heekerens, J. B., & Heinitz, K. (2019). Looking forward: The effect of the best-possible-self intervention on thriving through relative intrinsic goal pursuits. *Journal of Happiness Studies, 20*(5), 1379–1395. https://doi.org/10.1007/s10902-018-9999-6

Heinemann, L. V., & Heinemann, T. (2017). Burnout research: Emergence and scientific investigation of a contested diagnosis. *SAGE Open, 7*(1). https://doi.org/10.1177/2158244017697154

Hicken, M. T., Lee, H., Morenoff, J., House, J. S., & Williams, D. R. (2019). Racial/ethnic disparities in hypertension prevalence. Reconsidering the role of chronic stress. *American Journal of Public Health, 104*(1), 117–123.

Hutchinson, E. O. (1997). *The assassination of the Black male image*. Simon and Schuster.

Isaacs, J., Sawhill, I., & Haskins, R. (2007). *Getting ahead or losing ground: Economic mobility in America*. The Brookings Institution.

James, S. A. (1994). John Henryism and the health of African-Americans. *Culture, Medicine and Psychiatry, 18*(2), 163–182.

James, S. A., Hartnett, S. A., & Kalsbeek, W. D. (1983). John Henryism and blood pressure differences among black men. *Journal of Behavioral Medicine, 6*(3), 259–278.

Kieffer, C. H. (1984). Citizen empowerment: A developmental perspective. *Prevention in Human Services, 3*(2–3), 9–36.

Kirkinis, K., Pieterse, A. L., Martin, C., Agiliga, A., & Brownell, A. (2018). Racism, racial discrimination, and trauma: A systematic review of the social science literature. *Ethnicity & Health, 26*(3), 392–412.

Kottke, T. E., Stiefel, M., & Pronk, N. P. (2016). "Well-being in all policies": Promoting cross-sectoral collaboration to improve people's lives. *Preventing Chronic Disease, 13*, 1–7.

Krieger, N. (2020). ENOUGH: COVID-19, structural racism, police brutality, plutocracy, climate change—And time for health justice, democratic governance, and an equitable, sustainable future. *American Journal of Public Health, 110*(11), 1620–1623. https://ajph.aphapublications.org/doi/full/10.2105/AJPH.2020.305886

Kwate, N. O. A., & Meyer, I. H. (2010). The myth of meritocracy and African American health. *American Journal of Public Health, 100*(10), 1831–1834. https://doi.org/10.2105/ajph.2009.186445

Levinson, D. J. (1986). A conception of adult development. *American Psychologist, 41*(1), 3.

Martin, L. A., Neighbors, H. W., & Griffith, D. M. (2013). The experience of symptoms of depression in men vs women: Analysis of the National Comorbidity Survey Replication. *JAMA Psychiatry, 70*(10), 1100–1106.

McLeod, J. D. (2012). The meanings of stress: Expanding the stress process model. *Society and Mental Health, 2*(3), 172–186.

Mental Health America. (2021). *Covid-19 and mental health: A growing crisis*. Mental Health America.

Miller, C., & Vittrup, B. (2020). The indirect effects of police racial bias on African American families. *Journal of Family Issues, 41*(10), 1699–1722.

Mills, C. W. (2000). *The sociological imagination*. Oxford University Press.

Morgan, R., Baker, P., Griffith, D. M., Klein, S. L., Logie, C. H., Mwiine, A. A., Scheim, A. I., Shapiro, J. R., Smith, J., Wenham, C., & White, A. (2021). Beyond a zero-sum game: How does the impact of COVID-19 vary by gender? [Review]. *Frontiers in Sociology, 6*. https://doi.org/10.3389/fsoc.2021.650729

Morales, C. (2021). What we know about the shooting of Jacob Blake. The New York Times. https://www.nytimes.com/article/jacob-blake-shooting-kenosha.html#:~:text=Jacob%20Blake%2C%20a%2029%2Dyear,23%2C%202020.

National Academies of Sciences, Engineering, & Medicine. (2020). *Leading health indicators 2030: Advancing health, equity, and well-being*. The National Academies Press. https://doi.org/10.17226/25682

National Institute of Mental Health. (2017). *Men & depression*. https://www.nimh.nih.gov/health/publications/men-and-depression/index.shtml

National Institute of Mental Health. (2021). *About self-care*. Retrieved 2/1/2022 from https://www.nimh.nih.gov/health/topics/caring-for-your-mental-health

National Research Council. (2015). *Investing in the health and well-being of young adults*. National Academic Press.

Neighbors, H. W., Jackson, J. S., Broman, C., & Thompson, E. (1996). Racism and the mental health of African Americans: The role of self and system blame. *Ethnicity & Disease, 6*(1–2), 167–175.

Obama, M. (2021). *Becoming*. Crown.

Parker, L. J., Hunte, H., Ohmit, A., Furr-Holden, D., & Thorpe, R. J., Jr. (2017). The effects of discrimination are associated with cigarette smoking among black males. *Substance Use & Misuse, 52*(3), 383–391.

Pew Research Center. (2016). *Mobile fact sheet*. http://www.pewinternet.org/fact-sheet/mobile/.

Pieterse, A. L., & Carter, R. T. (2007). An examination of the relationship between general life stress, racism-related stress, and psychological health among Black men. *Journal of Counseling Psychology, 54*(1), 101–109.

Pittman, D. M., Brooks, J. J., Kaur, P., & Obasi, E. M. (2019). The cost of minority stress: Risky alcohol use and coping-motivated drinking behavior in African American college students. *Journal of Ethnicity in Substance Abuse, 18*(2), 257–278.

Poteat, T., Millett, G. A., Nelson, L. E., & Beyrer, C. (2020). Understanding COVID-19 risks and vulnerabilities among black communities in America: The lethal force of syndemics. *Annals of Epidemiology, 47*, 1–3.

Robert Wood Johnson Foundation. (2019). *Advancing well-being in an inequitable world: Moving from measurement to action* (Summary of insights from the Robert Wood Johnson Foundation's global conference on well-being, issue.) https://www.rwjf.org/en/library/research/2019/01/advancing-well-being-in-an-inequitable-world.html

Ruxton, S., & Burrell, S. (2020). *Masculinities and COVID-19: Making the connections*. Promundo-US.

Ryan, R. M., & Deci, E. L. (2000). Self-determination theory and the facilitation of intrinsic motivation, social development, and well-being. *American Psychologist, 55*(1), 68–78.

Seligman, M. E. P. (2011). *Flourish: A visionary new understanding of happiness and well-being*. Free Press.

Settersten, R. A., Jr., Ottusch, T. M., & Schneider, B. (2015). Becoming adult: Meanings of markers to adulthood. In *Emerging trends in the social and behavioral sciences: An interdisciplinary, searchable, and linkable resource* (pp. 1–16). Wiley.

Sherman, J. (2020). Dom Smith's pain shows how far away US is from racial justice. New York Post. https://nypost.com/2020/08/27/dom-smiths-pain-shows-how-far-away-us-is-from-racial-justice-sherman/

Singer, J., Sussman, N., Martin, N., & Johnson, A. (2020). *Black men have the shortest lifespans of any Americans. This theory helps explain why*. ProPublica. Retrieved 2/1/2022 from https://www.propublica.org/article/black-men-have-the-shortest-lifespans-of-any-americans-this-theory-helps-explain-why

Smith, J. A., Griffith, D. M., White, A., Baker, P., Watkins, D. C., Drummond, M., & Semlow, A. R. (2020a). COVID-19, equity and men's health: Using evidence to inform future public health policy, practice and research responses to pandemics. *International Journal of Men's Social and Community Health, 3*(1), e48–e64.

Smith, J. A., Watkins, D. C., & Griffith, D. M. (2020b). Equity, gender and health: New directions for global men's health promotion. *Health Promotion Journal of Australia, 31*(2), 161–165.

Stroud, C., Walker, L. R., Davis, M., & Irwin, C. E., Jr. (2015). Investing in the health and well-being of young adults. *Journal of Adolescent Health, 56*(2), 127–129.

Summers, M. A. (2004). *Manliness and its discontents: The Black middle class and the transformation of masculinity, 1900–1930*. University of North Carolina Press.

Summers, M. (2013). Manhood rights in the age of Jim Crow: Evaluating end-of-men claims in the context of African American history. *Boston University Law Review, 93*, 745–767.

Watkins, D. C. (2012). Depression over the adult life course for African American men: Toward a framework for research and practice. *American Journal of Men's Health, 6*(3), 194–210. https://doi.org/10.1177/1557988311424072

Watkins, D. C., & Neighbors, H. W. (2007). An initial exploration of what mental health means to young Black men. *The Journal of Men's Health & Gender, 4*(3), 271–282.

Watkins, D. C., Walker, R. L., & Griffith, D. M. (2010). A meta-study of Black male mental health and well-being. *Journal of Black Psychology, 36*(3), 303–330.

Watkins, D. C., Goodwill, J. R., Johnson, N. C., Casanova, A., Wei, T., Allen, J. O., Williams, E.-D. G., Anyiwo, N., Jackson, Z. A., Talley, L. M., & Abelson, J. M. (2020). An online behavioral health intervention promoting mental health, manhood, and social support for young Black men: The YBMen project. *American Journal of Men's Health, 14*(4), 1–17. https://doi.org/10.1177/1557988320937215

Watts, R. J., & Hipolito-Delgado, C. P. (2015). Thinking ourselves to liberation?: Advancing socio-political action in critical consciousness. *The Urban Review, 47*(5), 847–867. https://doi.org/10.1007/s11256-015-0341-x

Watts, R. J., Griffith, D. M., & Abdul-Adil, J. (1999). Socio-political development as an antidote for oppression. *American Journal of Community Psychology, 27*(2), 255–271.

Watts, R. J., Williams, N. C., & Jagers, R. J. (2003). Socio-political development. *American Journal of Community Psychology, 31*(1–2), 185–194.

Weitzer, R., & Brunson, R. K. (2015). Policing different racial groups in the United States. *Cahiers Politiestudies, 6*(35), 129.

Wheaton, F. V., Thomas, C. S., Roman, C., & Abdou, C. M. (2018). Discrimination and depressive symptoms among African American men across the adult lifecourse. *The Journals of Gerontology: Series B, 73*(2), 208–218.

Williams, D. R. (2003). The health of men: Structured inequalities and opportunities. *American Journal of Public Health, 93*(5), 724–731.

Williams, D. R., & Cooper, L. A. (2020). COVID-19 and health equity—A new kind of "herd immunity". *Journal of the American Medical Association, 323*(24), 2478–2480.

Williams, D. R., & Rucker, T. D. (2000). Understanding and addressing racial disparities in health care. *Health Care Financing Review, 21*(4), 75–90.

World Health Organization. (1946). *Preamble to the Constitution of the World Health Organization as adopted by the International Health Conference, New York, 19–22 June, 1946; signed on 22 July 1946 by the representatives of 61 States (Official Records of the World Health Organization, no. 2, p. 100) and entered into force on 7 April 1948.* World Health Organization. Retrieved January 9, 2017.

World Health Organization. (1986). Ottawa charter for health promotion, 1986. World Health Organization Regional Office for Europe.

World Health Organization. (2019). *Burn-out an "occupational phenomenon": International Classification of Diseases.* World Health Organization. Retrieved 2/1/2022 from https://www.who.int/news/item/28-05-2019-burn-out-an-occupational-phenomenon-international-classification-of-diseases.

Young Jr, A. A. (2017). The character assassination of black males: Some consequences for research in public health. In National Academies of Sciences (Eds.), Communities in action: Pathways to health equity (pp. 41–56). : National Academies Press.

Chapter 3
A Community-Based Ecosystems Approach for Promoting the Health, Wellbeing and Healing of Boys and Young Men of Colour

Phyllis Shu Hubbard

Why We Need a Community-Based Ecosystems Approach

In his thesis, Dr. Baloyi "redefines psychology and psychotherapy from the viewpoint of the African experience" (Baloyi, 2008, p. 1). He asserts that "the dominant Western paradigm of scientific knowledge in general and, psychology in particular, is anchored in a defective claim to neutrality, objectivity and universality because it obstructs Indigenous and pluriversal strategies for healing." This assertion is crucial to accurately supporting the need for a community-based ecosystems approach to promoting the health, wellbeing and healing of Boys and Young Men of Colour (BYMOC). Of equal importance is the necessity of addressing trauma specific to BYMOC by including healing strategies that can be substantiated through unconventional qualitative methodologies.

At the Association of Black Psychologists 50th anniversary convention, I surveyed the work of Dr. Baloyi and other psychologists of the African diaspora. They grappled with ways to promote and share their research to facilitate healing in Black communities. As I discovered that these challenges repeatedly surfaced during Black, Indigenous and Pacific islander convenings, I decided to infuse their research into my work with BYMOC populations.

P. S. Hubbard (✉)
Radiant Health Strategies, Oakland, CA, USA
e-mail: heal@phyllishubbard.com

My enthusiasm for helping children to realize their potential began as a teen mentor. During the summer I spent tutoring a young Black male, I discovered that emotional trauma was the root cause of his academic challenges (Harvey, 1996). Since that time, I have worked with BYMOC communities in various capacities, including talent recruitment, mentorship, and wellness training. My collaboration with the Campaign for Black Male Achievement (CBMA)[1] began in 2009, when I was invited to be a keynote speaker at their Transformational Leadership retreat. I created an interactive experience for the retreat called "Transformational Leadership from the Inside Out,"[2] based on strategies (for healing the mind, body, emotions, and spirit) that could be used to improve the personal and professional lives of its grantees. Although CBMA asked me to focus the presentation on nutrition, I firmly asserted that it was important to address unresolved emotional trauma (Carroll et al., 2021) and present it as a deep underlying root cause which, unless properly processed, would sabotage the success of BYMOC leaders and prevent them from thriving.

My affirmation is based on my research and personal experience. I was seven years old when I witnessed a traumatic event.[3] Shortly thereafter, I developed

---

[1] The Campaign for Black Male Achievement (CBMA) was an organisation focused on improving the life outcomes of leaders in the field of Black Male Achievement (BMA), which included community organisations and school personnel who mentored or educated Black males. Although the organisation focused its efforts primarily on BMA leaders, it funded and developed several programs that directly served Black males and BYMOC communities. CBMA ceased operations of the organization in December of 2020. The Black Male Achievement (BMA) Health and Healing Strategies and Journey to Radiance content is archived at https://www.phyllishubbard.com/community-collaborations, which serves as a community partner, radiant health advocate and role model to share, archive and preserve its content to ensure that the health and healing information is available for open source use globally.

[2] Dr. Phyllis Shu Hubbard created Transformational Leadership from the Inside Out as a theory of change model based on Radiant Health Strategies for self-mastery, self-empowerment, and active engagement in self-care.

[3] [When she was a child], Dr. Hubbard accidentally stumbled upon a preteen White boy raping a five-year-old Black girl. She immediately wanted to rush in to help but felt some force that froze her in place. She was confused by the White boy, who seemed to be talking aloud to no one and then realized, to her horror, that he was communicating with six Black boys who were watching the scene from a distance with their hands down their pants. The White boy was giving the Black boys instructions on how to rape the little girl. Though the boys had not yet spotted Dr. Hubbard, they were dangerously close. She realized that she had to make a quick exit to prevent herself from being attacked. She experienced a severe asthma attack as she attempted to explain to an adult what happened and then passed out before she could speak.

chronic obstructive pulmonary disease (COPD),[4] an incurable respiratory illness. After 27 years of enduring the negative side effects of prescription medication, I discovered that true healing lay in my ability to take care of myself in between doctor visits. I began to practice an ancient Indigenous form of medicine called Ayurveda which, when translated into English, means "the science of living."[5] The Ayurvedic remedies prompted the processing of suppressed and repressed emotions and mental health into its healing strategies. Within three months, my 27-year bout with COPD came to an end. This experience convinced me of the need to acknowledge and diligently work to heal trauma, inspiring me to study holistic health[6] and become an advocate for Radiant Health Strategies.[7]

---

[4] The COPD Foundation defines Chronic Obstructive Pulmonary Disease (COPD) as "chronic lung diseases including emphysema and chronic bronchitis. This disease is characterized by breathlessness. COPD is (currently) an incurable disease, but with the right diagnosis and treatment, there are many things you can do to breathe better and enjoy life and live for many years." (Source: https://www.copdfoundation.org/What-is-COPD/Understanding-COPD/What-is-COPD.aspx). Although the COPD Foundation considers COPD to be incurable, holistic health asserts that diseases are actually dis-eases (a lack of ease or balance in the body). For example, Ayurveda (defined in footnote number six) teaches that there are six stages of dis-ease, and that a person can reverse the course of dis-ease by identifying and removing the mental, emotional and physical root causes. Dr. Hubbard was on prescription medication which caused the COPD to become progressively worse. Ayurveda teaches that dis-ease originates as an emotion that, if not processed properly, weakens the body and makes it vulnerable to dis-ease. According to Ayurveda, if a person's *sadness, depression, guilt* and/or *grief* is suppressed, repressed and/or unhealed, it will cause a weakness or vulnerability in the *lungs*. This weakness is greatly exacerbated by the onset of a traumatic event. After practicing Ayurveda for three months, Dr. Hubbard's chronic cough stopped and she was able to reverse the course of the dis-ease.

[5] Ayurveda is an East Indian form of medicine that helps a person understand the profound effects that the mind and emotions have on the body. It uses self-awareness to help a person understand the difference between a balanced and imbalanced state. This increased level of awareness helps a person to make corrections and establish a heightened state of wellbeing regardless of illness or age. The practice of Ayurveda includes but is not limited to: elemental theory (the notion that the elements of ether, air, fire, water and earth are the building blocks and foundation of life for the body and for the universe); strategies for healing the body, mind, emotions and spirit; developing a wellness lifestyle; techniques for creating and/or re-establishing balance through setting and enforcing healthy boundaries, healing a person's emotions, the use of therapeutic nutrition and movement, herbal remedies, etc.

[6] Dr. Hubbard defines Holistic Health as a wellness lifestyle approach to healing that seeks to discover and correct imbalances in the person's physical body (including mental, emotional and spiritual health) and their social environment. Her Holistic Health expertise includes Ayurveda, Naturopathy (a system of healing that uses food, water, herbs, therapeutic massage and other physical therapeutic processes to facilitate the body's self-healing mechanisms), Kamitic/Kemetic (Ancient Egyptian) Yoga, Qigong (an ancient Chinese system of healing), Reiki (ancient Japanese system of energy healing), holistic nutrition and movement, aromatherapy, herbology, self-empowerment and cultural competency.

[7] Dr. Hubbard coined the term "Radiant Health Strategies" to promote healing of the body, mind, spirit and emotions so profound that it "radiates" wellness from one person to another and motivates people to inspire others to actively engage in self-care.

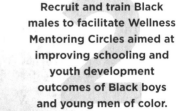

Provide caregivers
of children with
healing-centered
engagement strategies.

Recruit and train Black
males to facilitate Wellness
Mentoring Circles aimed at
improving schooling and
youth development
outcomes of Black boys
and young men of color.

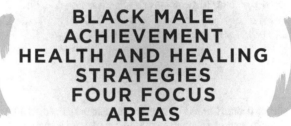

BLACK MALE
ACHIEVEMENT
HEALTH AND HEALING
STRATEGIES
FOUR FOCUS
AREAS

Provide resources for
strategic communication toward
asset-based narrative change
to guide members on how
to increase healthy and
healing lifestyles for
themselves and the young
men they serve.

Implement culturally
responsive teacher training
and professional development
designed to improve
classroom
management and reduce
stress for school personnel
and caregivers.

Fig. 3.1 Indicates BMA HHS' four primary focus areas

In 2016, The California Endowment[8] awarded a \$one million grant to CBMA for a health initiative within the Oakland and Sacramento City Unified School Districts, hiring Dr. Hubbard to create a program entitled Black Male Achievement (BMA) Health and Healing Strategies (HHS). She based BMA HHS on her research and conviction that the BYMOC field needs the support of a healthy ecosystem to succeed, grow and fulfil its potential. BMA HHS's focus areas included building the knowledge and skill sets needed to improve the physical and emotional health and overall wellness of the ecosystem of BYMOC (see Fig. 3.1).

---

[8] "California Endowment is a not-for-profit foundation with \$3.4 billion assets under management. The foundation primarily focuses on healthcare issues including access to health care, and health and well-being in California. It was founded in 1996 and is based in Los Angeles, California. Additional regional offices are situated in Sacramento, Fresno, San Diego, and Oakland." (Source: https://www.linkedin.com/company/the-california-endowment/). Learn more about the California Endowment at: https://www.calendow.org/

Building a Healthy Ecosystem

CBMA hosted a BMA HHS planning retreat with 34 school and community leaders to co-create a solid implementation strategy for the BMA HHS initiative in Northern California. The planning cohort decided to focus its efforts on supporting the psychosocial academic framework developed for middle and high school populations within Oakland Unified School District's African American Male Achievement Program (primarily Black males) and Sacramento City Unified School District's Men's Leadership Academy (BYMOC).

The team of trusted partners who lead the implementation of BMA HHS included Oakland and Sacramento City school districts and organizations working on behalf of BYMOC populations:

- Oakland Unified School District (which included some school personnel from San Francisco Unified School District)
- Sacramento City Unified School District
- National CARES Mentoring Movement
- Radiant Health Strategies
- Strategic Destiny, LLC
- 393Films
- A Touch of Life Leadership and Wellness Institute
- Flourish Agenda
- Spearitwurx

Oakland Unified School District's (OUSD's) Office of Equity addresses disproportionality for Black boys by employing a targeted-universal approach. Through the African American Male Achievement Initiative (AAMA) and the Manhood Development Program (MDP),[9] OUSD's efforts increase the grade point averages and reading levels of the African American male student program participants.[10] OUSD's Office of Equity creates systems change based on leveraging relationships and empowering people to challenge and radically disrupt oppressive systems. AAMA

---

[9] The Office of African American Male Achievement (AAMA) functions within the Oakland Unified School District (OUSD). OUSD was the first school district in the United States to create an office to address disproportionality amongst African American males. AAMA's Manhood Development Program is "a unique academic mentoring model designed and implemented *by* African American males *for* African American males. Instructors for the program were carefully chosen based upon cultural competency, understanding of youth development, and past experience teaching." (Source: https://www.ousd.org/Page/17777)

[10] Research data for OUSD AAMA and MDP student success can be found at: http://www.ousd-data.org/

(working in collaboration with the Kingmakers of Oakland[11]) was a vital partner in the implementation of BMA HHS in the City of Oakland. The subsequent section provides snapshots of the different activities implemented through BMA HHS. Specifically, the BMA HHS integration within OUSD included:

- CARES Mentoring Wellness Circles into OUSD's MDP[12]
- BMA HHS workshops during the OUSD Fall Forum and Spring Symposium[13]
- BMA HHS workshops during the Black Teacher Leadership and Sustainability Support Institute[14]
- BMA HHS workshops for community engagement events

One AAMA administrator reported that "MDP facilitators are beginning to remember/use the concepts; very positive reception to the info cards for home and classroom … [we need] more resources like this."

---

[11] After more than ten years in the district, a non-profit organization was developed called "Kingmakers of Oakland" (https://kingmakersofoakland.org/). Under the direction of Chris Chatmon (former Deputy Chief of OUSD's AAMA), "the independent non-profit now supports school districts across the country to improve the educational and life outcomes of Black boys by 'healing the fish while treating the toxic ecosystem.' This multi-faceted approach is rooted in a desire to collaborate, coordinate and convene folks who are inspired to create a healthy, affirming learning environment for Black boys in the public school system. Through professional development, narrative change, resources, curriculum and more, Kingmakers helps each unique district transform their school environment." (Source: https://kingmakersofoakland.org/who-we-are/story/)

[12] The National CARES Mentoring Movement is a pioneering, community-galvanizing movement, dedicated to alleviating intergenerational poverty among African Americans. It offers Black children in low-income families and underserved communities the social, emotional and academic support needed to unleash their potential and graduate from high school prepared to succeed in college or vocational-training programs and twenty-first century careers. More than 140,000 mentors and local CARES Affiliate Leaders across 58 U.S. cities are devoted to advancing young people who are often isolated and mostly written off by society. (Source: www.caresmentoring.org)

[13] "The OUSD Fall Forum [and Spring Symposium] is a multi-day conference showcasing the Kingmakers of Oakland model for African American Male Achievement. This event is an opportunity for participants to learn ways to address the systems, structures, conditions, and cultures that can lead to improved educational outcomes for African American boys from Pre-K to 12th grade. Participants will leave with an action plan to inspire leadership for Black boys in their own city, town, or region. The Fall Forum and Spring Symposium convene teams of students, teachers, principals, staff, administrators, and elected officials from a combination of school district, nonprofits, philanthropic and other educational institutions. The event is hosted each year by Kingmakers of Oakland, in collaboration with the African American Male Achievement Program within OUSD, as well as with their fiscal sponsor, The National Equity Project. (Source: https://kingmakersofoakland.org/event/fall-forum-2/)

[14] "The Black Teacher Leadership and Sustainability Institute is the Black Teacher Project's signature professional development offering – an experiential institute providing ample opportunities for Black teachers to share, reflect and set intentions for how to lead from the classroom. Teachers will deepen their commitment, relationships and agency while developing strategies for leadership and sustainability." (Source: https://www.blackteacherproject.org/)

Sacramento City Unified School District (SCUSD) provides targeted academic and social-emotional interventions offered through their Youth Development Support Services (YDSS). Programs include the Men's Leadership Academy (MLA)[15] and site-based, out-of-school-time opportunities (after-school and summer programs) that have increased school connectedness, attendance and high school graduation rates. Explicit in their goal to dismantle the school-to-prison pipeline and create systems to support the whole needs of the child and family, staff members of SCUSD's YDSS department were ideal partners for the implementation of BMA HHS in Sacramento City.

Sacramento City Unified School District (SCUSD)'s YDSS Department employs a social justice youth development framework toward empowering young men and women to be scholars of advocacy for self, culture and community. BMA Health and Healing Strategies offerings included:

- CARES Mentoring Wellness Circles at Sam Brannan Middle School and Will C. Wood Middle School
- BMA HHS workshops for district school personnel, community partners, families, and service providers
- A series of health and wellness challenges with district staff including fitness competitions, the creation of healthy work environments and offering healing-centred retreats

National CARES Mentoring Movement is a pioneering, community-galvanizing endeavour to offer Black children and underserved communities the social, emotional and academic support needed to unleash their potential and graduate from high school prepared to succeed in college or vocational-training programs and twenty-first century careers. More than 140,000 mentors and local CARES affiliate leaders across 58 U.S. cities are devoted to advancing young people who are often isolated and mostly written off by society.

BMA HHS collaborated with CARES Mentoring to elevate education, expectation, and self-esteem by engaging youth in community wellness circles. The CARES Mentoring Wellness Circles were implemented across five middle school sites in a partnership between Oakland Unified School District's Office of Equity and

---

[15] The Men's Leadership Academy is "a class offered during the school day (and for elective credit) to teens at risk of dropping out. Through service learning and a multicultural curriculum, the class aims to provide students with the tools to succeed, including teamwork, leadership, life skills, problem-solving and resiliency skills. The Academy focuses on bringing together teachers, students, parents and community businesses and partners to provide the encouragement needed for these teens to complete high school and enroll in college. The targeted audience for the Men's Leadership Academy is boys in grades 9–12 who have multiple risk factors, including low attendance, low academic performance and high suspension rates. Schools that have academies include C.K. McClatchy, John F. Kennedy, Rosemont, Arthur A. Benjamin Health Professions, American Legion and Sutter and California middle schools." (Source: https://www.scusd.edu/district-program/mens-leadership-academy)

Sacramento City Unified School District's Men's Leadership Academy (MLA). One mentee at Sam Brannan Middle School in Sacramento reported "I used to get into trouble with my teachers, now my grades are up." Another mentee shared that participating in mentoring circles "made me feel more responsible and helped me to think about life choices." The CARES Mentoring partners recruited and trained 240 adult mentors in Oakland and Sacramento, conducting 71 wellness mentoring sessions with a total of 440 youth participants.

Radiant Health Strategies (RHS), is a Holistic Health Education business, founded by Dr. Phyllis Shu Hubbard. RHS specializes in organizational, professional and personal transformation, sustainability, therapeutic nutrition and movement, clinical aromatherapy, herbalism, self-empowerment and cultural competency. Dr. Hubbard travels nationally and internationally as a holistic health educator, gathering research on Indigenous health practices to integrate into her healing techniques. RHS has provided customized wellness education for corporate and community organizations since 2007.

RHS launched BMA HHS and strategic communication endeavours, including recruiting 393Films[16] as a partner to co-host and produce the "Journey to Radiance" podcast and webisodes, facilitating transformational leadership workshops, producing numerous blogs, instructional videos and empowering images.[17] RHS encouraged BYMOC participants to discover their unique gifts and talents and actively engage in self-care through self-empowerment and wellness education. One workshop participant reported, "After leaving Dr. Hubbard's session, I made a vow to become better holistically. I changed my diet, started exercising and found a circle of friends to help hold me accountable." RHS facilitated 10 transformational leadership workshops, produced 27 blogs and educational posts and executive-produced and co-hosted 13 "Journey to Radiance" podcasts, two "Journey to Radiance" webisodes, and a "Journey to Radiance" theme song.

Strategic Destiny: Designing Futures Through Faith and Facts was founded by Reverend Dr. Alfonso Wyatt. Strategic Destiny seeks to find common language and

---

[16] 393Films is a Bay Area-based full production house that specializes in screenwriting, directing and editing with state-of-the-art equipment and innovative digital media software. 393Films creates multimedia projects that inspires action. Founder Adimu Madyun has an extensive history of production and service. An educator, filmmaker, and musician, Adimu, a.k.a. "WolfHawkJaguar," has produced films and music in both the United States and various African countries. Additionally, he facilitates the DetermiNation Black Men's Group, a men of color achievement circle (through partnership with United Roots and Urban Peace Movement) and trains youth in media and music production. (Source: www.393films.com and www.unitedrootsoakland.org)

[17] The Journey to Radiance podcast and webisodes aimed to promote healthy lifestyles, share empowering healing strategies and provide accurate, positive and healthy depictions of Black men and boys, specifically as it relates to cultural identity, health and healing. Dr. Phyllis Shu Hubbard (Radiant Health Strategies) and WolfHawkJaguar (393Films) served as co-hosts and producers of the Journey To Radiance multimedia series. The "Journey to Radiance" theme song and multimedia productions are available for open-source use to the public at: https://www.phyllishubbard. com/community-collaborations

collaborative opportunities with socially engaged practitioners who are motivated by faith, as well as secular practitioners motivated by evidence-based learning. Through workshops, training and healing circle facilitation, Strategic Destiny empowers caregivers to support their own healing and to influence the health and wellness of the youth they serve. Dr. Wyatt is a renowned national speaker on issues affecting men, children, youth, adults, families, community mental and physical health. In his role as a national public theologian, he offers a message of hope in and out of the faith community. Dr. Wyatt provides consulting to government institutions, universities, foundations, public/charter schools, non-profits and civic groups.

In alignment with BMA HHS, Strategic Destiny provided workshops and training to community-based organizations, educators and families. SCUSD YDSS collaborated with Dr. Wyatt to provide crisis-response support and community healing for Sacramento families, district staff and community members after the tragic loss of Stephon Clark, a young Black man killed by police in March of 2018.[18]

One Strategic Destiny workshop participant reported that they learned "tools for reframing and redirecting student behavior and using strength-based language." Strategic Destiny facilitated 11 workshops with a total of 328 participants.[19]

393Films creates multimedia projects aimed at transforming thoughts through creating media that inspires action. A San Francisco (USA) Bay Area-based full production house, 393Films' services include screenwriting, directing and editing with state-of-the-art equipment and innovative digital media software. Founder Adimu Madyun, a.k.a. "WolfHawkJaguar," has an extensive history of production and service. An educator, filmmaker and musician, Adimu has produced films and music in both the United States and various African countries. Additionally, he

---

[18] "In the late evening of March 18, 2018, Stephon Clark, a 22-year-old African-American man, was shot and killed in Meadowview, Sacramento City, California by Terrence Mercadal and Jared Robinet, two officers of the Sacramento City Police Department in the backyard of his grandmother's house while he had a phone in his hand. The encounter was filmed by police video cameras and by a Sacramento City County Sheriff's Department helicopter which was involved in observing Clark on the ground and in directing ground officers to the point at which the shooting took place. The officers stated that they shot Clark, firing 20 rounds, believing that he had pointed a gun at them. Police found only a cell phone on him. While the Sacramento City County Coroner's autopsy report concluded that Clark was shot seven times, including three shots to the right side of the back, the pathologist hired by the Clark family stated that Clark was shot eight times, including six times in the back. The shooting caused large protests in Sacramento City, and Clark's family members have rejected the initial police description of the events leading to Clark's death. The Sacramento City Police Department placed the officers on paid administrative leave and opened a use of force investigation. Police have stated they are confident that Clark was the suspect responsible for breaking windows in the area prior to the encounter." (Source: https://en.wikipedia.org/wiki/Shooting_of_Stephon_Clark)

[19] The Strategic Destiny workshops offered extensive follow-up (including handouts and take-home activities). Some presentations were facilitated as a series. Although each workshop welcomed new attendees, the total may include duplicate participants who attended more than one session.

facilitates the DetermiNation Black Men's Group and trains youth in media and music production.[20]

In partnership with BMA HHS, 393Films co-hosted and produced the "Journey to Radiance" podcast to shift the narrative around BYMOC, specifically as it related to health and healing. The overarching goal for this collaboration was to elevate accurate, positive, and healthy lifestyles of BYMOC. An activist, who calls himself "Young Black Soul," left the following review of "Journey to Radiance": "This is a great podcast! Journey to Radiance focuses on one of the most pervasive issues in the Black community–Health and Healing. Learn more about the art of health and healing through this high quality, informative, podcast! Side-note: awesome intro track!" Another reviewer shared, "I can't recommend this podcast enough. Much needed and happy you're creating this for us! Thank you." 393Films produced 13 "Journey to Radiance" podcasts, two "Journey to Radiance" Webisodes, and a "Journey to Radiance" theme song which was written by Dr. Hubbard and edited, performed and produced by Adimu Madyun.

A Touch of Life is a health and wellness institute that specializes in facilitating transformational teambuilding and employee wellness training for non-profit organizations, corporations and county/state institutions. Founder Asara Tsehai brings more than 35 years of experience in the health and wellness industry to her training and workshops. Ms. Tsehai's work has been featured in several national publications, including *Essence, Sister to Sister* and *Heart and Soul* magazines. A Touch of Life provided BMA HHS sessions to Oakland Unified School District's MDP personnel. Session topics included overall health and wellbeing, nutrition, reflexology, yoga, and guided development of individualized personal wellness plans. One wellness session participant reported that Asara's sessions "created space to recharge/re-energize and ground one-self." Another participant shared that "[I'm] shifting patterns of

---

[20]The DetermiNation Black Men's Group is a program developed by United Roots of Oakland, a Youth Impact Hub. "United Roots, in partnership with Urban Peace Movement, launched the DetermiNation youth program in May 2013. DetermiNation is a program designed to support the success and development of young African American males (ages 16–24) from the Oakland area (the DetermiNation project was created and developed by Markese Bryant of Fight for Light). The DetermiNation program is especially tailored to support young men who are struggling to advance in their own life goals (such as employment, career, educational, or other personal goals) and who have been formerly involved in or are currently in close proximity to the "street life." As part of the program, youth participants will develop their media production skills and produce projects like short films, music and graphic design to share their personal stories and/or present a vision of what is possible for young men of color in our communities. The media production will be part of the Boys and Men of Color media engagement strategy (a statewide initiative led by The California Endowment: https://www.calendow.org/). DetermiNation was developed by Markese Bryant (CEO of Flight for Light), and the lead facilitator is Adimu Madyun (393Films). The program entails a weekly support group for young Black males, with opportunities to do media production with youth groups throughout California. Participants will learn about Black culture and history and develop new skills and tools for achieving life goals. The program will also offer basic instruction in media production, and participants will be required to produce media projects as part of the training. Participants will receive a stipend for participation in weekly training sessions and have the opportunity for additional paid opportunities doing media production. For more information go to: www.DetermiNationMedia.org (Source: https://www.unitedrootsoakland.org/determination.html)

behaviour (workaholic mode, over exertion), toward a more meditative state." A Touch of Life facilitated a total of 20 workshop sessions for the 25 OUSD MDP staff members.

Flourish Agenda is a national non-profit consulting firm that works with youth of colour, schools, youth serving organizations, foundations, and local governments to build and implement strategies that allow young people to flourish. They are the leading providers of the healing-centred engagement strategies, tools and research that are necessary to reimagine how systems can more effectively support young people of colour.[21] Flourish Agenda's mission is to design strategies that unlock the power of healing and engage youth of colour and adults in transforming their schools and communities. Their healing-centred engagement approach is a non-clinical and holistic process involving culture, spirituality, civic action, and collective healing. It views trauma not simply as an individual isolated experience, but rather highlights the ways in which trauma and healing are experienced collectively. The term "healing-centred engagement" expands how participants think about responses to trauma and offers a more holistic approach to fostering well-being.

Flourish Agenda conducted seminars, workshops and trainings with K-12 teachers, non-traditional educators, and district staff in each of the two targeted communities in Oakland and Sacramento City. Their Healing-Centred Engagement workshops in schools and communities included strategies to support personal self-care, healing, and tools toward the integration of a healing-centred approach in educational practices. Additional BMA HHS efforts included:

- Keynote addresses by Founder, author and CEO Dr. Shawn Ginwright
- Healing Centered Engagement workshops and retreats that provide breakthrough experiences to educational practitioners and caregivers
- Customized services to support institutions and evaluate program impact and effectiveness
- Application of research findings on youth of color, racial trauma and well-being to improve practices and inform the field

Flourish Agenda facilitated 13 sessions with a total of 309 participants.[22] More than 80% of participants reported being motivated and willing to use the Healing-Centred Engagement model for their youth and for their personal enrichment. Some

---

[21] "Healing Centered Engagement is an asset-based and culturally-rooted approach to healing and well-being for young people of color and their adult allies. The term was coined by Dr. Shawn Ginwright in 2018 and is based on more than 30 years of research and practice with young people, schools, probation departments and social workers." (Source: https://flourishagenda.com/healing-centered-engagement-certification/). The healing centered engagement approach is a non-clinical and holistic process involving culture, spirituality, civic action and collective healing. It views trauma not simply as an individual isolated experience, but rather highlights the ways in which trauma and healing are experienced collectively.

[22] Flourish Agenda workshops offered extensive follow-up (including handouts and take-home activities). Some presentations were facilitated as a series. Although each workshop welcomed new attendees, the total may include duplicate participants who attended more than one session.

participants were already using the model and enthusiastically attended these popular workshops as a refresher to their previous training experiences.

Spearitwurx provides innovative consulting and training for parents and youth development professionals on topics such as powerful parenting, staff wellness and sustainability, crisis intervention, intergenerational and vicarious trauma, classroom management, restorative justice, effective team building and more. Spearitwurx's mission is to develop young people's ability to actively contribute to the transformation of their families and create a healthy and sustainable community. They fulfil their mission by equipping youth development professionals with the right tools to engage and empower youth toward health and wellness. Additionally, Spearitwurx focuses on building support within families to provide a safe space for parents and youth to share strategies on how to build safety, sustainability, and solidarity.

In alignment with BMA HHS, Spearitwurx provided monthly healing-centred workshops for parents, families, and community members within the Oakland Unified School District. Most notably, at West Oakland Middle School, Spearitwurx bridged the cultural gap between the school community's African American and Yemeni families through engagement in shared health and healing learning opportunities for parents and guardians. One participant shared, "If the parents felt welcomed and loved in schools, we would be able to do so much more for the children." Spearitwurx facilitated 10 sessions with a total of 362 participants.[23]

BMA HHS Participant Engagement

Since its official launch in Spring of 2016, BMA HHS engaged 2436 youth, educators, school district personnel, parents/guardians, youth practitioners and community members in various opportunities designed to build transformative leadership and promote health, healing, and overall wellness for BYMOC, including, but not limited to, the following:

- Facilitation of more than 135 health and healing workshops, seminars and retreats
- Engagement of 440 middle school boys in wellness mentoring circles
- Production of 13 BMA HHS podcasts and 2 webisodes containing health and healing demonstrations, an affirmative theme song and numerous educational graphics (see Fig. 3.2)
- Recruitment and training of 240 mentors
- Facilitation of informational workshops and caregiver retreats with 354 parents, grandparents and/or guardians
- Development of 27 BMA health and healings blogs and educational posts

---

[23] Spearitwurx workshops offered extensive follow-up (including handouts and take-home activities). Some presentations were facilitated as a series. Although each workshop welcomed new attendees, the total may include duplicate participants who attended more than one session.

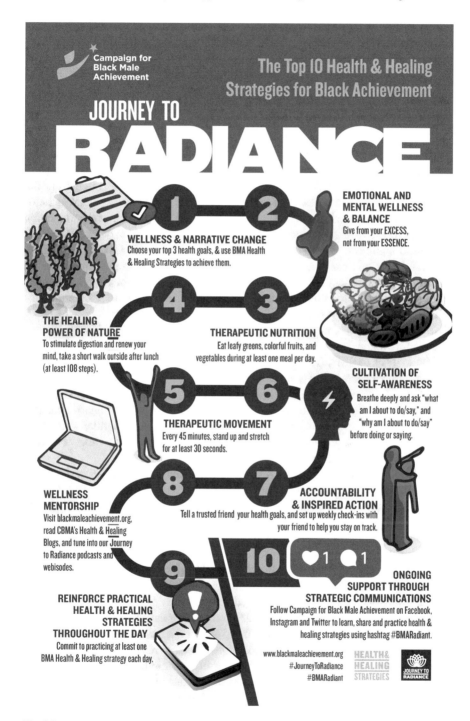

Fig. 3.2 An example of BMA HHS educational graphics provided to the public

Ninety-one percent of workshop participants were motivated to increase physical activity; and 82% of workshop participants learned new skills to help reduce the negative effects of stress and trauma.

Evaluation and Methodology

During the second year of the initiative, Dr. Hubbard engaged a local evaluation partner, Innovation Bridge, to capture, document and analyse impact. The following sections detail the methodology and key findings of that assessment. Historically, the BYMOC community has often found itself the subject of research that pathologized negative narratives, yielding more harm than benefits for the community. Repeated research-related atrocities have harmed, silenced and exploited BYMOC, leading to significant distrust between researchers and the BYMOC community. Understanding this context, this methodology sought to "illuminate the complex dimensions of goodness" (Lawrence-Lightfoot & Davis, 1997, p. xvi) as a counterpoint to the dominant culture and tradition of documenting failure in communities of colour. The overall goal was to capture the wholeness and complexity of BMA HHS as it related to structures, people, relationships, goals, education, and voice. The section below details how data was collected and evaluated.

The analysis of BMA HHS commenced at the start of the second year. Innovation Bridge collected data using workshop attendance, post-workshop provider surveys and informal interviews with stakeholders to capture impact during the first year of implementation. The team surveyed attendance to provide a preliminary quantitative outlook on engagement and participation in the various programs and workshops, and reviewed post-workshop surveys and stakeholder interviews to obtain preliminary qualitative data.

The evaluation team began primary data collection during the second year of implementation. This data centred on participant evaluation surveys and field observations. The objective was to ascertain the impact and sustainability of health and healing strategies within participants' everyday lifestyle and practices. Innovation Bridge conducted field observations to gain a better understanding of participant-level impact. The team conducted their observations from the vantage point of participant observers, who attended the full breadth of programming while on site, taking intermittent notes. Innovation Bridge then debriefed and expanded on the notes.

The evaluation team analysed targeted data via document review and provider focus groups to verify and support initial findings from the preliminary data review. Analysis of provider focus groups conducted during the second year of implementation and document review data, in conjunction with the primary data, provided additional clarity. The team and strategic partner organizations facilitated participant focus groups to further understand the impact of strategies on youth, practitioners, and families. Innovation Bridge examined and triangulated the data for impact themes through the three data profiles (primary, targeted and analysis; see Fig. 3.3).

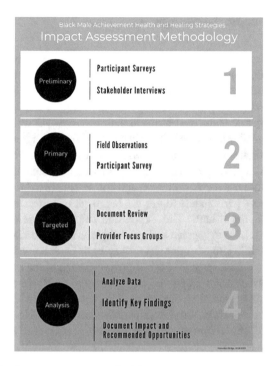

Fig. 3.3 Illustrating impact assessment methodology

The team identified and cross-referenced emerging themes with health and heal-ing strategies for relevance. They shared a preliminary write-up of the findings with BMA partners, who provided additional clarity and feedback. The feedback was used as an additional analytical tool to determine the overall impact, giving voice to the community to capture the "complex dimensions of goodness" associated with BMA HHS. Innovation Bridge organized their findings based on effective BMA HHS strategies, key opportunities and recommendations moving forward.

Fostering a Community-Based Ecosystems Approach

The information that follows summarizes the most impactful Health and Healing Strategies within the implementation and evaluation of this initiative. The evalua-tion team highlighted practices that may be useful for individuals looking to begin or enhance their personal journey to wellness, offering suggestions for those who support others on their paths to health and healing.

Confirming Specific Language

The first key finding from BMA HHS was the power of affirmative language in the healing process. This included both the acquisition and understanding of supportive language. One of the barriers to healing is the inability to name what is wrong and to address the need for healing. Learning the "language of self-care" enabled participants to identify and name the trauma in their own lives, as well as in the lives of BYMOC. Additionally, it allowed participants to refine the identification of their emotions and facilitate better communication, youth-to-youth, youth-to-adult, and adult-to-adult, in the process of securing empowering and authentic relationships.

The CARES wellness mentors created and consistently used memorable slogans to encourage student participants to use the language of self-care. One example is the expression "Saying it Out." This expression empowered students to articulate their feelings, learn how to receive and respond to critical feedback and feel more confident in their ability to communicate. "Saying it Out" helped students provide counter statements, or ask questions for improved clarity, to maintain balance when emotionally triggered, which improved engagement in their schoolwork.

Flourish Agenda provided teachers and school personnel with the language of CARMA – Culture, Agency, Relationships, Meaning and Aspirations (Ginwright, 2016). As one of the Flourish Agenda session participants stated, "Through CARMA, I have been able to attune and refine the abstract attitudes and behaviors that no longer serve me." For this participant, acquiring the language has not only led to an evaluation of the behaviors that serve them, but has supported them in building healthy relationships as they engage in therapy and liberation work in the community. Acquiring the word "agency" helped another participant to identify toxic relationships and take control of one's mental health. CARMA provided clarity of purpose and improved her sense of confidence and personal power.

Flourish Agenda addressed their youth participants as "wellness contributors" and community "change agents." This reframing shifted limiting beliefs about BYMOC as they developed spiritual practices, growth mindsets and healthy ways of living which made a positive impression on adults, particularly as the youth discovered their identity and purpose.

Creating Safe Spaces

The cultivation of safe healing spaces is another strategy that showed evidence of impact across BMA HHS partners and participants. Adult participants described their experiences of working within the school systems as "high stress, non-affirming and littered with microaggressions." Youth participants spoke of school as a place that constantly threatened their physical and social-emotional safety. They also described having to endure fights, excessive discipline, low achievement, and a lack of confidence. The BMA HHS partners worked diligently to curate peaceful meeting spaces and infuse Indigenous healing circle rituals (Mehl-Madrona &

Mainguy, 2014) into their sessions.[24] The BMA HHS participants considered the meeting spaces to be places of refuge and healing for people of colour. The attendees obtained valuable problem-solving and stress-management skills that they could explore with their colleagues and apply to novel situations.

Dr. Alfonso Wyatt of Strategic Destiny communicated the importance of cultivating a familial connection with his participants. Because there were grandparents raising their grandchildren who participated in his workshops, he worked to find spaces within the community of the attendees to create an increased sense of safety, comfort and convenience.

Allowing Permission for Self-Care and Wellness Practices

Many BMA HHS partners stressed the importance of working with school personnel and community leaders to allow permission for, promote and prioritize self-care. This foundation allowed participants to remix their approach to building relationships with BYMOC. Claudette Lee and Ethel Williams stated that "survival … racism, discrimination and oppression define the childhood of an African American male" (2001, p. 56). This narrative can often be interpreted through the lens of fear for the survival of BYMOC, leading caring adults to inadvertently approach relationship building through the vehicle of toughness, aggression or hypermasculinity.

The mothers and grandmothers who participated in the BMA HHS workshop sessions led by Spearitwurx spoke about the fear that comes from the challenge of raising BYMOC in Oakland, CA. Yet, as part of their BMA HHS efforts, Spearitwurx emphasized the importance of self-care as a process of dealing with the increasing stressors of raising BYMOC. They recommended strategies such as "connecting before you correct," and "taking a breath before you engage in the correction process to make it more meaningful and less punitive." These more thoughtful approaches to correction impacted how the participants of Spearitwurx engaged with their children. As one participant stated, the strategies she's learned have helped her to "not be so aggressive" and to "calm myself down" when communicating with her grandchildren. Other participants noted that, despite the view that you can't "slack on your mack with town teenagers," the strategies of "more love and hugs, reciprocity with positivity," and being more open to learning how to communicate with their children/grandchildren led to positive change.

---

[24] "[Indigenous] Healing circles … consist of people who sit together in a talking circle, in prayer, in ceremony, and are committed to helping one another and to each other's healing." (Source: https://www.ncbi.nlm.nih.gov/pmc/articles/PMC4022550/). BMA HHS Indigenous healing circle rituals would often include burning sage, palo santo or another traditional incense to clean the energy of the room before attendees arrive/during the opening ceremony, setting boundaries and intentions at the beginning of the session, taking a few moments to acknowledge the ancestors, the use of a talking piece such as a healing crystal or stone, breathing exercises with movement, engaging the participants in simple art projects to express their feelings, icebreaker games to set or change a mood, etc.

Engaging Intergenerational Role Models

One of the most prominent areas of impact was the interactive engagement of inter-generational role models (youth, adults and elders). The CARES mentors noted that the students who participated in their wellness circles at both the Oakland and Sacramento City sites experienced improved grades, confidence, behaviour and communication skills. Student focus group participants reported that the wellness circle sessions were a protected space that allowed them to express their emotions in healthy ways. Participating in the wellness circles increased their awareness and personal responsibility to self and community, including modelling respectful and positive male-female relationships. Utilizing intergenerational role models to demonstrate and empower youth to create counter-narratives resulted in academic and interpersonal success. One middle school principal noted, "The boys have learned how to forgive each other."

The intergenerational role models consistently affirmed the BYMOC participants with empowering titles to focus them on a vision for their success. Spearitwurx presented BYMOC as "entrepreneurs," providing place and space for students to be seen as resources to their community through their pop-up resource village. Spearitwurx also employed a catering company founded by a 13-year-old African American male to provide healthy food for their workshops.

Additional Factors to Consider

The following recommendations are focused more specifically on challenges and opportunities to increase BMA HHS for BYMOC within educational, city and community-based systems of support. Several BMA HHS partners noted the complexity and challenges of promoting wellness within the various school systems. These obstacles impacted their access to a diversity of potential participants who could benefit from their programming. The strategic partners asserted the need for school-wide and district-wide buy-in from institutional partners, as well as an emphasis on streamlining access to space and potential participants for effective implementation.

While participants from educational systems spoke to the value and safety of having spaces that were primarily for people of colour, there was also an acknowledgment that it was important to engage their White peers in the process. Attendees reported a dire need for motivating white staff and educational leaders to participate in the process of self-care and to improve cultural competence to facilitate narrative change and the creation of a healthy ecosystem for BYMOC in schools.

Although background checks are used to contribute to the overall safety of schools, they can also serve as a barrier to the inclusion and participation of male adults of colour. Though the culture of mass incarceration and the prison-industrial

complex[25] disproportionately impacts men of colour, this fact is not addressed within the current policies around background checks, specifically regarding schools and/or youth-serving organizations. Consequently, males of colour are frequently excluded from program leadership. Unfortunately, access to health and healing strategies that can assist BYMOC in recovering from trauma experienced within the justice system (through direct and/or indirect involvement) is denied due to their association with those justice systems. BMA HHS partners and participants noted how the work is incomplete and, in some ways, self-defeating if these opportunities for participation continue to be elusive for men of colour.

Recognizing that the specific health and healing needs for BYMOC in each city, school district and community are unique, how can we build on impactful strategies from Northern California to expand the work of this initiative to other communities throughout the country? What online or web-based opportunities exist for learning collaborations between Oakland or Sacramento City and other cities like Detroit, Michigan where BMA HHS work has commenced? Furthermore, how do we expand to more explicitly address the critical needs of BYMOC, such as nutritional and mental health needs at various stages of life, or health and healing support for BYMOC who are gender non-conforming, non-binary or transgender?

References

Baloyi, L. (2008). Psychology and psychotherapy redefined from the viewpoint of the African experience. In *Doctoral dissertation, November 2008*. University of South Africa.

Carroll, A., York, A., Fynes-Clinton, S., et al. (2021). The downstream effects of teacher Well-being programs: Improvements in teachers' stress, cognition and Well-being benefit their students. *Frontiers in Psychology, 12*, 689628. https://doi.org/10.3389/fpsyg.2021.689628

Ginwright, S. (2016). *Hope and healing in urban education: How urban activists and teachers are reclaiming matters of the heart*. Routledge.

Harvey, M. R. (1996). An ecological view of psychological trauma and trauma recovery. *Journal of Traumatic Stress, 9*(1), 3–23.

Lawrence-Lightfoot, S., & Davis, J. H. (1997). *The art and science of portraiture*. Jossey-Bass.

Lee, C., & Williams, E. H. (2001). Masculinity, matriarchy and myth: A black feminist perspective. In A. O'Reilly (Ed.), *Mothers and sons: Feminism, masculinity, and the struggle to raise our sons* (pp. 56–68). Routledge.

Mehl-Madrona, L., & Mainguy, B. (2014). Introducing healing circles and talking circles into primary care. *The Permanente Journal, 18*(2), 4–9. https://doi.org/10.7812/TPP/13-104

---

[25] The prison-industrial complex is a term that makes the connection between various prisons systems (such as juvenile detention centers, prisons, psychiatric hospitals, etc.) and the businesses/government that financially benefit from their growth and expansion.

Chapter 4
First-Generation Black College Men in the United States and the Value of Cohort-Based Programs: Addressing Inequities Through the YBMen Project

Daphne C. Watkins, Brittany Ribeiro Brown, Jamie M. Abelson, and James Ellis

Introduction

Though many Black men enrolled in college encounter conflict, resistance, and alienation (Howard et al., 2012; Thayer, 2000), researchers are beginning to distinguish the experiences of first-generation Black college men (FG-BCM – that is, students whose parents did not attend college) from continuing-generation Black college men (CG-BCM, that is students whose parents attended college). For instance, compared to men whose parents attended college, FG-BCM report feeling like they do not belong, that they lack motivation (to complete their degree) and that they face challenges with the college transition, particularly in light of a heightened racial climate in U.S. colleges and universities (Hoffman et al., 2002; Locks et al., 2008; Owens et al., 2010). Participating in cohort-based programs and practices significantly improves success, removes barriers, and builds and sustains a community for first-generation college students (Charleston & Leon, 2016; Engle & Tinto, 2008). Furthermore, FG-BCM benefit significantly from cohort programs (Ellis & Helaire, 2018; McGowan & Pérez, 2020; Taylor, 2018) such that their sense of belonging, health, wellbeing, and graduation rates improve (Douglas & Attewell, 2014). There is a need for more programs that enhance the health and academic performance of FG-BCM. Given the different experiences FG-BCM face on the way to and through college compared to their continuing-generation counterparts, evidence-based programs have the potential to leverage the strengths FG-BCM bring with them to college toward a promising future.

D. C. Watkins (✉) · B. R. Brown · J. M. Abelson · J. Ellis
School of Social Work, University of Michigan–Ann Arbor, Ann Arbor, MI, USA
e-mail: daphnew@umich.edu; bnrb@umich.edu; jabel@umich.edu; jmelli@umich.edu

© The Editor(s) (if applicable) and The Author(s), under exclusive license to 53
Springer Nature Switzerland AG 2023
J. A. Smith et al. (eds.), *Health Promotion with Adolescent Boys and Young Men of Colour*, https://doi.org/10.1007/978-3-031-22174-3_4

The Young Black Men, Masculinities, and Mental Health (YBMen) project launched in 2014 as a social media-based psychoeducation program for Black men. The YBMen intervention uses gender-specific, age-appropriate, and culturally sensitive popular culture (e.g., songs, movies, sports, GIFs, YouTube, and news headlines) to educate participants about mental health, progressive masculine norms, and social support. To date, we have delivered the YBMen intervention to over 300 Black men across five college and university campuses in the U.S. Midwest. The YBMen Project has been successful in decreasing depressive symptoms, expanding masculine norms, and increasing social support for Black college men (Goodwill et al., 2018; Goodwill et al., 2019; Watkins, 2019; Watkins et al., 2017; Watkins et al., 2020). Previous iterations of the YBMen intervention have achieved the program outcomes for both FG and CG Black college men (Watkins et al., 2020). The purpose of this chapter is to discuss the inherent value of the YBMen project in addressing inequities in mental health (i.e., outcomes, stigma, literacy), social support, and social capital for FG-BCM.

Background and Literature Review

First-Generation College Students

Increased access to higher education over the past 40 years has increased the number of high school students who aspire to attend college. For instance, the number of high school students enrolling in college upon graduation increased from 63% in 2000 to 70% in 2016 (National Center for Education Statistics, 2020). These aspiring college students are the first in their immediate families to attend college. These "first-generation college students" make up approximately one-third of all college attendees, including two-year and four-year colleges (Anderson, 2017). First-generation college students often come from lower socioeconomic backgrounds. They may experience barriers in their pursuit of a college degree, such as lacking the information needed to select a school, completing a college application, navigating the financial aid application process, and gathering the social capital necessary for a positive college experience (Ward et al., 2012). This is in addition to the academic expectations and demands needed to maintain high grade point averages and acquire the necessary information to complete a college degree.

Even after controlling for family income and academic preparation, parental college degree attainment remains a significant factor in student persistence and degree completion (Choy, 2001). Previous studies underscore the challenges first-generation students face, compared to their continuing-generation counterparts, such as accessing, financing, and completing their degrees (Stephens et al., 2012). First-generation college students receive less assistance in preparing for college and may not be as academically well-prepared as students whose parents attended college. They also tend to experience less support from family members who are unfamiliar with the collegiate experience. Additionally, first-generation college students negotiate between meeting family obligations, such as caring for younger siblings, and meeting their academic obligations (Covarrubias & Fryberg, 2015; Vasquez-Salgado et al., 2015). Given the need to remain connected to their families and communities back home, first-generation students may also lack a sense of belonging to the institution they attend. But the pull away from the college experience extends beyond activities back home, as many first-generation college students tend to live off-campus and work more hours per week than continuing-education students (Strand, 2013). These experiences do not worsen the college experience for first-generation students; however, they translate into different experiences for first-generation students compared with continuing-education students.

Forty-two percent of continuing-generation college students graduate in four years, while only 27% of first-generation students graduate during that time frame (Cataldi et al., 2018; DeAngelo et al., 2011). First-generation college students are more likely to take longer to graduate: 50% of them graduate within six years (DeAngelo et al., 2011). While the number of first-generation college students enrolled at colleges and universities across the U.S. is increasing (Inkelas et al., 2007), the number of first-generation college graduates is not increasing. Also, given the academic adjustments and alterations to college applications made during the 2020-'21 pandemic, higher education should anticipate more first-generation students entering college post-pandemic in hopes of improving their conditions and that of their families and communities. Furthermore, colleges and universities will look to first-generation college students to maintain their enrolment numbers (Krantz, 2018) and ensure that these students persist in the coming years, as the need for more leaders will increase to get the economy back on track from the economic and political recession experienced during the 2020-'21 pandemic. While the number of students applying for college has declined overall during the pandemic, we anticipate that the number will increase over time.

Colleges and universities have dedicated institutional resources such as academic advising, tutoring, mentoring, peer instruction, and small learning communities to help retain students of colour, including first-generation college students of colour. However, efforts to identify which assets and personal attributes of first-generation students result in their persistence and successful college completion are sparse (Thayer, 2000). Also, the various elements that contribute to the success of first-generation college students have been discussed in the literature (Blackwell & Pinder, 2014; Naumann et al., 2003; Petty, 2014; Próspero et al., 2012), yet these studies are limited in scope and methods; they use either quantitative or qualitative methods, and tend to focus on a single attribute that contributes to the overall success of first-generation students.

Black College Students

College enrollment for Black students has increased over the past 40 years. For example, 10% of undergraduate students were Black in 1980 compared to 13.2% in 2018. Despite the steady increase in Black college students, Black college women have consistently outnumbered Black college men 2:1 (Perry, 2009). Black college students frequently face stressors related to the campus climate and institution type, which can ultimately shape and significantly impact their academic performance, wellbeing, and overall college experience (Greer & Brown, 2011; Mincey et al., 2014; Oliver et al., 2017; Womack & Sloan, 2017).

Studies that measure Black college students' health status are usually conducted on a single campus, assessing Black college men and women's health, with women primarily oversampled (Lundy-Wagner & Gasman, 2011). Furthermore, Black students may enter college having already experienced stressors related to financial difficulty and college readiness (Banks, 2010; Greer et al., 2015; Greer & Brown, 2011; Hu & Wolniak, 2013). Employment is also a common stressor for Black college students, as they sometimes need to work to pay tuition (Watkins et al., 2007) and to alleviate some of the financial strains on their loved ones back home (Wood et al., 2011). The added responsibility of working to support oneself and one's immediate or extended family members contributes to adverse psychosocial health outcomes for Black college students who are simultaneously learning to navigate the rigorous academic demands of their college lives. It also makes it challenging for them to fully engage in the college experience and reap the rewards.

Much of our knowledge about Black college students' health comes from historically Black colleges/universities (HBCUs) (Mushonga & Henneberger, 2020). Although the number of studies conducted with Black college students is growing, prior research with this group has been limited due to the sampling methodologies used and the absence of students who attended non-HBCUs. Similarly, findings are mixed in determining academic outcomes and emotional wellbeing among students enrolled at HBCUs compared to those enrolled at predominantly white institutions (PWIs). For example, Black students enrolled at HBCUs have reported better academic outcomes (e.g., higher GPA, retention rates, and graduation rates), more positive relationships with faculty, more robust social networks and friendships, and have higher rates of overall satisfaction (Patton et al., 2011; Seifert et al., 2006). However, other studies found no significant differences between Black students at HBCUs and Black students at PWIs when exploring these outcomes (Flores & Park, 2015).

In addition to the differences in campus climate, being a first-generation college student, having negative interactions with White faculty, and experiencing racial discrimination on campus have all been identified as stressors germane to Black college students (Blackmon et al., 2016; Ellis et al., 2015; Greer & Brown, 2011; Guiffrida & Douthit, 2010; Jones & Greene, 2016; Kohn-Wood et al., 2012). Researchers would be remiss to overlook chronic stressors nested within race and racism, as activism on college campuses has increased since the tumultuous events surrounding recent social justice issues— notably, Black Lives Matter (Hope et al., 2016), and the aftermath of George Floyd's and Breonna Taylor's deaths.

Black College Men

Mental Health Outcomes and Stigma

The percentage of Black men ages 18-to-24 who enrolled in college increased from 25% to 33% between 2000 and 2018, respectively (Hussar et al., 2020). Recent national data from the *Healthy Minds Study* found Black men make up 5% of all college students, and 34% of those Black male students reported experiencing depression, anxiety, an eating disorder, any non-suicidal self-injury, or any suicidal ideation over the past year (Lipson et al., 2018). Despite their mental health challenges, only 23% of Black college men use psychotropic medication or therapy. In comparison, 59% prefer informal help-seeking from family and friends and cohort-based (e.g., race/gender-focused) programs.

The complexity of disorders such as depression, as it manifests across race, culture, and gender norms, presents a multi-layered phenomenon for Black men (Watkins, 2012). The aetiology and symptomatology of mental disorders are influenced by the complex nature of being both Black and male, making it difficult to diagnose, treat, and monitor a race and gendered phenomenon such as depression. Despite the complexity of depression for Black men, several studies have attempted to understand the factors that lead to depression and depressive symptoms for Black college men (Barry et al., 2016; Watkins, 2012; Watkins et al., 2006; Watkins et al., 2007; Watkins & Neighbors, 2007).

Mental health stigma discourages students from self-disclosing mental health problems because doing so will result in bias and limit their professional development opportunities (Martin, 2010). Mental health stigma is associated with lower quality of life (Corrigan & Watson, 2002) and impedes access to education, income, healthcare, employment, and housing (Seroalo et al., 2014; Sharac et al., 2010). Mental health stigma is negatively associated with help-seeking attitudes among undergraduate students (Clement et al., 2015; Masuda & Boone, 2011) and their perceived need for treatment and other support (Eisenberg et al., 2009). Among college students, mental health stigma has been linked to increased psychological distress (Denenny et al., 2015; Goodwill & Zhou, 2020), exacerbated stress, depression, and suicidal behaviours (Hirsch et al., 2017). Yet, Black college men's mental health challenges have largely been left out of national conversations about college students' mental health. Furthermore, these conversations rarely occur in Black communities due to the stigma associated with mental health conditions. This barrier makes mental health challenges challenging to address. The structural racism and discrimination in healthcare also make it challenging to monitor Black college men's health as they transition to and through adulthood.

Mental Health Literacy

High mental health stigma and low mental health literacy have previously been reported among college men (Goodwill & Zhou, 2020; Rafal et al., 2018; Ratnayake & Hyde, 2019), and Black college men (Watkins et al., 2010; Watkins & Neighbors, 2007). Mental health illiteracy is a barrier to seeking and receiving quality mental health care and treatment for Black men (Watkins et al., 2010). To have confidence that it is worth seeking care, it is essential to know that (1) what one is experiencing is not rare and is treatable, (2) medications can work, (3) what kind of providers exist (e.g., social workers, psychologists, and psychiatrists), and (4) how to access them via school and the community. Traumatic events leave a mark, and Black college men need to know help is available. Given the current high suicide rates among Black youth, it is important to know that it is worth seeking help when one experiences suicidal thoughts or feelings. Mental health literacy also encompasses learning about actions that can protect one's mental health during stressful times.

Social Support

Existing research on the social support networks of Black men is limited and usually involves the relationships of socially and economically marginalised men, such as those involved in street life (Oliver, 2006; Payne, 2011), the criminal justice system (Gaines, 2007), homeless men (Littrell & Beck, 2001), and low-income non-residential fathers (Anderson et al., 2005). Despite these limitations in the research, it demonstrates that kinship and social support are essential for maintaining a sense of community and support for issues surrounding the health of Black men (Plowden et al., 2006; Plowden & Young, 2003). For example, Plowden and Young (2003) suggested that support networks' influence is a critical social factor in motivating their sample of urban Black men to seek health care and participate in health-related activities. The concept of support is vital to understanding Black men's social, behavioural, and mental health outcomes. Studies suggest Black college men report advantages to building strong relationships with their college peers (Brooms et al., 2015; Harper, 2013; McGowan, 2016; Strayhorn, 2008). Social support has also dominated focus group discussions with Black college men, particularly Black men at PWIs (Watkins et al., 2007). Other studies have identified peers as a significant influence on how young Black men define mental health and model their current and future health behaviours (Watkins, 2012; Watkins & Neighbors, 2007).

Social support among men has direct implications for social functioning. In more recent years, the use of online support groups and social media platforms has quadrupled (Ellison et al., 2014; Oh et al., 2014). The anonymity and confidentiality they offer increase the potential of self-disclosure and encourage honesty and intimacy among participants when discussing stigmatising health topics (Kernsmith & Kernsmith, 2008). Online support groups and social media platforms are typically self-help in nature, and studies have reported positive outcomes from their use, most notably in decreasing depression (Morgan & Cotton, 2003). Online communities and social media networks provide Black men with a 24/7 accessible space for communicating about topics that might be uncomfortable for face-to-face groups of Black men (e.g., stress, racism, etc.) (Watkins et al., 2017; Watkins & Jefferson, 2013). Another appealing feature of online groups and social media networks is that they are less spontaneous than face-to-face encounters, allowing participants to think about their responses before sharing them with other participants (Kernsmith & Kernsmith, 2008). Furthermore, men of all races who participate in online groups are more empathetic to the problems experienced by other men. All-male support groups do not often share this experience in face-to-face settings. Due to the COVID-19 pandemic, some men likely became even more familiar with online social connections than they were previously, which made connecting this way even more accessible than it was in the past.

Social Capital

Social capital is a combination of network size, relationship strength, and resources possessed by those in the group relative to its network and contact resources (Flap, 2004; Lin & Huang, 2005). *Network resources* are resources that an individual can access and include: (a) range among ties, distance; (b) reachability; (c) variety/heterogeneity; (d) and composition (Lin & Huang, 2005; Van Der Gaag & Snijders, 2005). *Contact resources* indicate valued resources represented by contacts or helpers in specific actions. The valued resources of the connection (e.g., wealth, power, status) positively affect job searches and career advances (Batistic & Tymon, 2017; Finsveen & Oorschot, 2008; Flap, 2004; Lin & Huang, 2005). The structure and scope of higher education support the development of social capital during the college experience. Students are provided an opportunity to develop bridging, bonding, accessible, and mobilised network connections.

Lack of social capital is often associated with first-generation student status. Social capital is a resource that one gains through relationships and interactions with others in one's social network, facilitating subsequent social and economic action (Coleman, 1988). First-generation students tend to have lower cultural and social capital than continuing generation students, leading to a general lack of knowledge about the college environment and lower self-efficacy (Pascarella et al., 2004; Soria & Stebleton, 2012). Generating social capital, such as wealth, power, and status, often from a college-educated parent, also leads to economic resources and opportunities such as internships and employment (Lin & Huang, 2005). Social capital leverages resources embedded in the social structure, accessibility to these social resources, and utilization or mobilization of social resources through purposive actions (Finsveen & Oorschot, 2008; Lin, 2001).

Previous research on social capital among Black college men at PWIs (Harper, 2008) and HBCUs (Palmer et al., 2009; Palmer & Gasman, 2008) focused on access to social capital networks, leadership positions, and involvement with clubs and organisations on campus. Students reported that their access to these networks helped them become informed about exclusive resources, scholarships, internships, and networking opportunities. However, this research has been limited in research methods (primarily qualitative) and scope (focused on the PWI vs. HBCU experience). College students reap benefits from social media to generate social capital, as Ellison et al. (2007) found strong associations between Facebook usage and social capital. In the subsequent sections, we will review the YBMen Project, discuss ways the YBMen Project can address inequities for FG-BCM, and discuss the implications for health promotion for FG-BCM in research, practice, and policy.

The YBMen Project

Intervention Description

The YBMen project is an evidence-based psychoeducation program launched in 2014 as a social media-based mental health education and social support intervention for Black men. The YBMen intervention uses gender-specific, age-appropriate, and culturally sensitive resources from popular culture (e.g., song lyrics, photos, YouTube videos, news headlines) to educate participants about the importance of mental health, progressive definitions of manhood, and social support (Watkins et al., 2017; Watkins et al., 2020). Since the intervention's inception, the social media platforms Facebook and Instagram have been used to reach young Black men with adapted program content. For each YBMen intervention, the team partners with communities and college campuses to adapt the curriculum with identified groups of Black men.

Curriculum Overview

The YBMen intervention is grounded in techniques focused on action planning and feedback, group problem-solving, and individual decision-making to achieve intervention outcomes. These techniques are expounded upon during each week's topic (See Fig. 4.1 for a sample YBMen intervention curriculum). This chapter demonstrates how the YBMen intervention curriculum can be adapted for FG-BCM. For example, during Module 1 (week 1), participants can be introduced to the YBMen group and oriented to the intervention style and format. They can also be presented with information about first-generation Black college students' experiences compared to continuing-generation students as a way to contextualize the purpose and objectives of subsequent intervention modules.

During Module 2 (weeks 2 through 5), participants can be introduced to depression, depressive symptoms, mental health stigma, mental health literacy, and the differences between clinical severity of mood disorders and stress. During Module 3 (weeks 6 and 7), participants can receive information about traditional masculine norms, Black masculinities, and the notion that multiple masculinities exist beyond rigidly defined gender roles. This idea is essential for FG-BCM as they may have

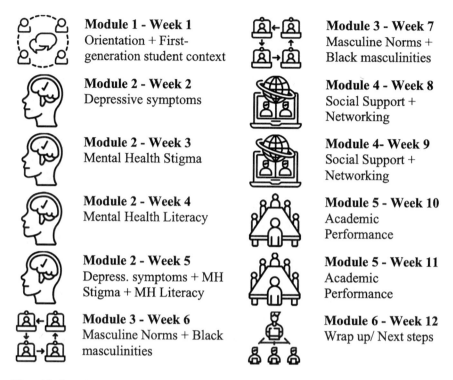

Fig. 4.1 Sample 12-Week YBMen Intervention Curriculum for First-Generation Black College Men

specific definitions of manhood that challenge the role of higher education in their lives. Module 4 (weeks 8 and 9) can cover the importance of social support, sustaining healthy social relationships, and social networking for FG-BCM.

Module 5 (weeks 10 and 11) can focus on academic performance for FG-BCM and how they can excel in college and beyond. For example, for FG-BCM, this module can contain content about various academic performance dimensions and review participants' educational practices and norms as college students. Module 6 (weeks 11 and 12) can review content from previous weeks and establish individual and group sustainability plans and help FG-BCM carry what was learned during the YBMen intervention into their remaining college years and beyond.

Addressing Inequities Through the YBMen Project for First-Generation Black college Men

Weekly themes and curriculum content can include a range of topics chosen by the partnering campus. For example, the social and racial injustices documented in the U.S. over the past few years have led to an expansion of our traditional YBMen intervention topics. Partnering communities and campuses now want to include content related to public safety, policing, and anti-racism in our standard YBMen intervention curriculum. The nature of the YBMen intervention curriculum is that every time the program is delivered, it is adapted to the specific population and time period (so it can respond to what is currently taking place for the participants). This means an adaptation stage is always built into the YBMen intervention, and curriculum enhancements are anticipated and embraced. The nature of YBMen is that it builds community, provides structure in which participants can be themselves, and offers psychoeducation on topics pertinent to Black men. Therefore, the YBMen Project is promising in addressing inequities in mental health (i.e., outcomes, stigma, literacy), social support, and social capital for FG-BCM compared to CG-BCM (Fig. 4.2).

Cohort-based health promotion interventions for Black college men that are culturally sensitive, age-appropriate, and gender-specific provide a unique opportunity to intervene when they are susceptible to stress, depression, and risky health behaviours that contribute to premature morbidity and mortality. Simultaneously, it remains challenging to engage Black college men in traditional health interventions; therefore, adapting and delivering online cohort-based psychoeducation programs is promising. As a group, Black men tend to report high rates of social media use (Watkins & Jefferson, 2013), and these rates have likely increased since the COVID-19 pandemic. Therefore, the YBMen intervention serves as a platform from which colleges and universities can enrich the mental health, definitions of masculine norms, and social support of FG-BCM. Not only does the evidence-based YBMen intervention achieve its primary outcomes, but it can also address previously described inequities in the college experience between FG-BCM compared to CG-BCM.

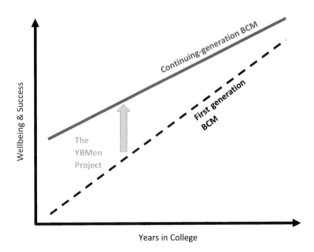

Fig. 4.2 The Potential for the YBMen Project to Address Inequities Between First-Generation and Continuing-Generation Black College Men

Implications for Promoting the Health of Boys and Young Men of Colour: Research, Practice, and Policy Considerations

As more first-generation college students enter higher education, implementing cohort-based programs helps to support their mental health, social support, and academic needs (House et al., 2020). Delivering the YBMen Project to FG-BCM will address inequities in mental health (i.e., outcomes, stigma, literacy), social support, and social capital experienced by FG-BCM compared to CG-BCM. A concerted effort has yet to occur that reduces inequalities in social capital for FG-BCM while simultaneously evaluating their response to an adapted, internet-based intervention that aims to improve their mental health, masculine norms, social support, and academic performance. Institutions must retain and graduate FG-BCM to identify the students most in need and develop programming to support them during their college experiences. This proactive approach will help improve retention rates of FG-BCM, allowing them to feel socially supported and attain better health, psychosocial adjustment, coping behaviours, quality of life, and self-actualisation (Watkins et al., 2017). More gender-specific, age-appropriate, and culturally sensitive programs are needed to improve the transitions and trajectories of FG-BCM. Cohort-based programs like the YBMen Project have and will continue to show promising results in closing the gaps reported between the experiences of FG and CG Black college men.

To date, we have conducted five pilot and efficacy trials with the YBMen Project across college and university campuses in Michigan and Ohio (USA). The project is currently being piloted with young Aboriginal and Torres Strait Islander males in the Northern Territory of Australia, and we hope to adapt a version of the program with African, Caribbean, and Black men in Toronto in the coming years. Our preliminary studies have determined that the YBMen intervention improves mental health (i.e., decreases depressive symptoms), expands masculine norms (i.e., gives participants a broader definition of manhood), and increases social support for Black college men. However, the intervention can do even more for FG-BCM. In particular, the YBMen intervention can reduce inequalities in social capital, reduce mental health stigma, increase mental health literacy, and improve academic performance for FG-BCM. Scaling the YBMen intervention to other sites serving first-generation men, both in the U.S. and around the globe, will fill a critical gap by reducing the inequalities associated with Black college men's first-generation status compared to continuing-generation students. Our preliminary studies of Black college men provide an essential lens to scale and sustain the YBMen Project for FG-BCM and show promise for impacting Black college men at research, practice, and policy levels.

At the *research* level, our previous findings suggest online interventions are beneficial for Black men (Watkins, 2019; Watkins & Jefferson, 2013) and that private social media groups are valuable mechanisms for delivering mental health education to Black college men. A report from our 2015 pilot with 18-to-25-year-old Black college men (n = 30) at a small, 2-year college in Michigan (Watkins et al.,

2017) showed that Black college men enjoyed the YBMen intervention's opportunities for relationship building and connectivity online. We also found that popular culture references encouraged Black college men to actively participate in the YBMen intervention (Watkins et al., 2017). Findings also supported previous studies (Chiang et al., 2004; Watkins et al., 2006), revealing that Black college men hold less favourable views towards counselling and rely heavily on informal support networks as their preferred coping strategy. Future research should focus on the experiences of FG-BCM compared to CG-BCM at HBCUs and PWIs. Mixed methods are a way to add the context of FG and CG Black college men's experiences to statistical measures of causation.

At the *practice* level, we have uncovered ways that Black college men cope with various stressors that impact their mental health (Goodwill et al., 2018). Several challenges surface when Black men's mental health is examined for research and practice purposes (Keating, 2009). Greater knowledge of risk and protective factors for FG-BCM can improve our understanding of the problems that lead to poor mental health and potentially severe disorders such as depression. More information is needed about FG-BCM's social, gendered, and behavioural health norms to better understand the experiences that shape their positive educational outcomes. In previous YBMen interventions, Black college men reported coping with stress by talking with members of their social support networks, engaging in physical activities (i.e., exercise), and relying on themselves. Some respondents said they intentionally avoided dealing with their mental health but noted the value in the cohort-based approach of the YBMen Project. Stigma emerged as a barrier to seeking help, and study findings highlighted within-group differences among Black college men. They also noted the importance of developing creative ways to examine stress and coping with culturally relevant and readily available resources both within and outside of spaces Black men occupy at the university (Goodwill et al., 2018). Future practice efforts should underscore the value of within-group differences among FG and CG Black college men and dedicate resources to ensure programming is in place to support the strengths that both groups bring to their college experiences.

At the *policy* level, there is promise and potential for how colleges and universities can institutionalize programming for FG-BCM. Now that we know Black college men value opportunities to discuss how various social determinants influence their mental health, colleges and universities should identify clear budget lines to support these programs. Cohort-based programs for first-generation Black college students that examine facets of their mental health, gender norms, social support, social capital, and academic performance are desperately needed. Similarly, a more in-depth, contextualized study of Black college students' experience by gender is sparse in the literature, despite researchers calling for a comprehensive investigation of Black college men's first-generation student experiences, apart from that of Black college women (Becerra, 2017). It is necessary for institutions facing the problem of retaining and graduating first-generation college students (1) to find ways of identifying the students most in need and (2) develop policies and programming to support them.

Conclusion

Though earlier YBMen iterations improved mental health, expanded masculine norms, and improved social support outcomes for Black male participants, recent YBMen interventions have included measures for first-generation student status. We have learned from previous research and YBMen data that the experiences of FG-BCM are different from that of CG-BCM. Building on our previous work, we believe adapting and scaling the YBMen Project will improve the lives of FG-BCM by decreasing their depressive symptoms and mental health stigma, increasing mental health literacy, expanding masculine norms, increasing social support, and improving social capital and their academic performance. This proactive approach – adapting and delivering the YBMen intervention as a unique cohort program for FG-BCM – enables colleges and universities to be more cost-effective and prudent in their expenditures on such student services. This will also help colleges and universities improve their recruitment and retention rates of Black college men, while simultaneously promoting the health and wellbeing of, and reducing the health inequities faced by, Black college men.

References

Anderson, N. (2017). A third of students applying to college via common app are first-gen. The Washington Post. https://www.washingtonpost.com/news/grade-point/wp/2017/10/20/a-third-of-students-applying-to-college-via-common-app-are-first-gen/

Anderson, E. A., Kohler, J. K., & Letiecq, B. L. (2005). Predictors of depression among low-income, nonresidential fathers. *Journal of Family Issues, 26*(5), 547–567. https://doi.org/10.1177/0192513X04272753

Banks, K. H. (2010). African American college students' experience of racial discrimination and the role of college hassles. *Journal of College Student Development, 51*(1), 23–34. https://doi.org/10.1353/csd.0.0115

Barry, A. E., Jackson, Z., Watkins, D. C., Goodwill, J. R., & Hunte, H. E. (2016). Alcohol use and mental health conditions among black college males: Do those attending postsecondary minority institutions fare better than those at primarily white institutions? *American Journal of Men's Health, 11*(4), 962–968. https://doi.org/10.1177/1557988316674840

Batistic, S., & Tymon, A. (2017). Networking behaviour, graduate employability: A social capital perspective. *Education + Training, 59*(4), 374–388. https://doi.org/10.1108/ET-06-2016-0100

Becerra, M. (2017). *Mental health and academic performance of first-generation college students and continuing-generation college students*. UC Merced Library. https://escholarship.org/uc/item/4691k02z

Blackmon, S. M., Coyle, L. D., Davenport, S., Owens, A. C., & Sparrow, C. (2016). Linking racial-ethnic socialization to culture and race-specific coping among African American college students. *Journal of Black Psychology, 42*(6), 549–576. https://doi.org/10.1177/0095798415617865

Blackwell, E., & Pinder, P. J. (2014). What are the motivational factors of first-generation minority college students who overcome their family histories to pursue higher education? *College Student Journal, 48*(1), 45–56.

Brooms, D. R., Goodman, J., & Clark, J. (2015). "We need more of this": Engaging black men on college campuses. *College Student Affairs Journal, 33*(1), 105–123. https://doi.org/10.1353/csj.2015.0002

Cataldi, E. F., Bennett, C. T., & Chen, X. (2018). First-generation students: College access, persistence, and postbachelor's outcomes. Stats in brief. NCES 2018-421. *National Center for education statistics.*

Charleston, L., & Leon, R. (2016). Constructing self-efficacy in STEM graduate education. *Journal for Multicultural Education, 10*(2), 152–166. https://doi.org/10.1108/JME-12-2015-0048

Chiang, L., Hunter, C. D., & Yeh, C. J. (2004). Coping attitudes, sources, and practices among black and Latino college students. *Adolescence, 39*(156), 793–815.

Choy, S. P. (2001). Students whose parents did not go to college: Postsecondary access, persistence, and attainment. *The condition of education, 16,* Washington DC: National Center for education statistics, xviii–xliii.

Clement, S., Schauman, O., Graham, T., Maggioni, F., Evans-Lacko, S., Bezborodovs, N., & Thornicroft, G. (2015). What is the impact of mental health-related stigma on help-seeking? A systematic review of quantitative and qualitative studies. *Psychological Medicine, 45*(1), 11–27. https://doi.org/10.1017/S0033291714000129

Coleman, J. S. (1988). Social capital in the creation of human capital. *American Journal of Sociology, 94,* S95–S121.

Corrigan, P. W., & Watson, A. C. (2002). Understanding the impact of stigma on people with mental illness. *World Psychiatry: Official Journal of the World Psychiatric Association, 1*(1), 16–20.

Covarrubias, R., & Fryberg, S. A. (2015). Movin' on up (to college): First-generation college students' experiences with family achievement guilt. *Cultural Diversity and Ethnic Minority Psychology, 21*(3), 420–429. https://doi.org/10.1037/a0037844

DeAngelo, L., Franke, R., Hurtado, S., Pryor, J. H., & Tran, S. (2011). *Completing college: Assessing graduation rates at four-year institutions.* Higher Education Research Institute, UCLA.

Denenny, D., Thompson, E., Pitts, S. C., Dixon, L. B., & Schiffman, J. (2015). Subthreshold psychotic symptom distress, self-stigma, and peer social support among college students with mental health concerns. *Psychiatric Rehabilitation Journal, 38*(2), 164–170. https://doi.org/10.1037/prj0000124

Douglas, D., & Attewell, P. (2014). The bridge and the troll underneath: Summer bridge programs and degree completion. *American Journal of Education, 121*(1), 87–109.

Eisenberg, D., Downs, M. F., Golberstein, E., & Zivin, K. (2009). Stigma and help seeking for mental health among college students. *Medical Care Res & Review, 66*(5), 522–541. https://doi.org/10.1177/1077558709335173

Ellis, J. M., & Helaire, L. J. (2018). The effects of adolescent self-regulated learning on engagement in a college access program: An exploratory study. *AERA Open, 4*(1), 1–17. https://doi.org/10.1177/2332858418756051

Ellis, J. M., Rowley, L. L., Nellum, C. J., & Smith, C. D. (2015). From alienation to efficacy: An examination of racial identity and racial academic stereotypes among black male adolescents. *Urban Education, 53*(7), 1–30. https://doi.org/10.1177/0042085915602538

Ellison, N. B., Steinfield, C., & Lampe, C. (2007). The benefits of Facebook "friends:" social capital and college students' use of online social network sites. *Journal of Computer-Mediated Communication, 12*(4), 1143–1168. https://doi.org/10.1111/j.1083-6101.2007.00367.x

Ellison, N. B., Vitak, J., Gray, R., & Lampe, C. (2014). Cultivating social resources on social network sites: Facebook relationship maintenance behaviors and their role in social capital processes. *Journal of Computer-Mediated Communication, 19*(4), 855–870. https://doi.org/10.1111/jcc4.12078

Engle, J., & Tinto, V. (2008). *Moving beyond access: College success for low-income, first-generation students.* Pell Institute for the Study of Opportunity in Higher Education. https://files.eric.ed.gov/fulltext/ED504448.pdf

Finsveen, E., & Oorschot, W. V. (2008). Access to resources in networks: A theoretical and empirical critique of networks as a proxy for social capital. *Acta Sociologica, 51*(4), 293–307. https://doi.org/10.1177/0001699308097375

Flap, H. (2004). Creation and returns of social capital: A new research program. In H. Flap & B. Völker (Eds.), *Creation and returns of social capital: A new research program (Vol. 9)* (pp. 2–17). Routledge.

Flores, S. M., & Park, T. J. (2015). The effect of enrolling in a minority-serving institution for black and Hispanic students in Texas. *Research in Higher Education, 56*(3), 247–276. https://doi.org/10.1007/s11162-014-9342-y

Gaines, J. S. (2007). Social correlates of psychological distress among adult African American males. *Journal of Black Studies, 37*(6), 827–858. https://doi.org/10.1177/0021934705285566

Goodwill, J. R., & Zhou, S. (2020). Association between perceived public stigma and suicidal behaviors among college students of color in the U.S. *Journal of Affective Disorders, 262*, 1–7. https://doi.org/10.1016/j.jad.2019.10.019

Goodwill, J. R., Watkins, D. C., Johnson, N. C., & Allen, J. O. (2018). An exploratory study of stress and coping among black college men. *American Journal of Orthopsychiatry, 88*(5), 538–549. https://doi.org/10.1037/ort0000313

Goodwill, J. R., Anyiwo, N., Williams, E. D. G., Johnson, N. C., Mattis, J. S., & Watkins, D. C. (2019). Media representations of popular culture figures and the construction of black masculinities. *Psychology of Men & Masculinities, 20*(3), 288–298. https://doi.org/10.1037/men0000164

Greer, T. M., & Brown, P. (2011). Minority status stress and coping processes among African American college students. *Journal of Diversity in Higher Education, 4*(1), 26–38. https://doi.org/10.1037/a0021267

Greer, T. M., Ricks, J., & Baylor, A. A. (2015). The moderating role of coping strategies in understanding the effects of intragroup race-related stressors on academic performance and overall levels of perceived stress for African American students. *Journal of Black Psychology, 41*(6), 565–585. https://doi.org/10.1177/0095798414560018

Guiffrida, D. A., & Douthit, K. Z. (2010). The Black student experience at predominantly White colleges: Implications for school and college 118 counsellors. *Journal of Counseling & Development, 88*(3), 311–318.

Harper, S. R. (2008). Realizing the intended outcomes of Brown: High-achieving African American male undergraduates and social capital. *American Behavioral Scientist, 51*(7), 1030–1053. https://doi.org/10.1177/0002764207312004

Harper, S. R. (2013). Am I my brother's teacher? Black undergraduates, racial socialization, and peer pedagogies in predominantly white postsecondary contexts. *Review of Research in Education, 37*(1), 183–211. https://doi.org/10.3102/0091732X12471300

Hirsch, J. K., Rabon, J. K., Reynolds, E. E., Barton, A. L., & Chang, E. C. (2017). Perceived stress and suicidal behaviors in college students: Conditional indirect effects of depressive symptoms and mental health stigma. *Stigma and Health, 4*(1), 98–106. https://doi.org/10.1037/sah0000125

Hoffman, M., Richmond, J., Morrow, J., & Salomone, K. (2002). Investigating "sense of belonging" in first-year college students. *Journal of College Student Retention: Research, Theory & Practice, 4*(3), 227–256.

Hope, E. C., Keels, M., & Durkee, M. I. (2016). Participation in black lives matter and deferred action for childhood arrivals: Modern activism among black and Latino college students. *Journal of Diversity in Higher Education, 9*(3), 203–215. https://doi.org/10.1037/dhe0000032

House, L. A., Neal, C., & Kolb, J. (2020). Supporting the mental health needs of first generation college students. *Journal of College Student Psychotherapy, 34*(2), 157–167.

Howard, T. C., Flennaugh, T. K., & Terry, C. L. (2012). Black males, social imagery, and the disruption of pathological identities: Implications for research and teaching. *Educational Foundations, 26*(1–2), 85–102.

Hu, S., & Wolniak, G. C. (2013). College student engagement and early career earnings: Differences by gender, race/ethnicity, and academic preparation. *The Review of Higher Education, 36*(2), 211–233.

Hussar, B., Zhang, J., Hein, S., Wang, K., Roberts, A., Cui, J., Smith, M., Bullock Mann, F., Barmer, A., & Dilig, R. (2020). The Condition of Education 2020. *NCES*, 2020144. https://nces.ed.gov/pubsearch/pubsinfo.asp?pubid=2020144

Inkelas, K. K., Daver, Z. E., Vogt, K. E., & Leonard, J. B. (2007). Living–learning programs and first-generation college students' academic and social transition to college. *Research in Higher Education, 48*(4), 403–434. https://doi.org/10.1007/s11162-006-9031-6

Jones, C. A., & Greene, H. T. (2016). Race discrimination, racial socialization, and offending trends among African American college students: A test of the theory of African American offending. *Journal of Contemporary Criminal Justice, 32*(1), 60–77. https://doi.org/10.1177/1043986215607255

Keating, F. (2009). African and Caribbean men and mental health. *Ethnicity and Inequalities in Health and Social Care, 2*(2), 41–53. https://doi.org/10.1108/17570980200900015

Kernsmith, P. D., & Kernsmith, R. M. (2008). A safe place for predators: Online treatment of recovering sex offenders. *Journal of Technology in Human Services, 26*(2–4), 223–238. https://doi.org/10.1080/15228830802096598

Kohn-Wood, L. P., Hammond, W. P., Haynes, T. F., Ferguson, K. K., & Jackson, B. A. (2012). Coping styles, depressive symptoms and race during the transition to adulthood. *Mental Health, Religion & Culture, 15*(4), 363–372. https://doi.org/10.1080/13674676.2011.577059

Krantz, L. (2018). New England colleges have one big worry: 2025. The Boston Globe. https://www.bostonglobe.com/metro/2018/02/03/new-england-colleges-have-one-big-worry/DWUWVTg36Z2Yz9C8QO9sAM/story.html

Lin, N. (2001). *Social capital: A theory of social structure and action*. Cambridge University Press.

Lin, S. C., & Huang, Y. M. (2005). The role of social capital in the relationship between human capital and career mobility: Moderator or mediator? *Journal of Intellectual Capital, 6*(2), 191–205. https://doi.org/10.1108/14691930510592799

Lipson, S. K., Kern, A., Eisenberg, D., & Breland-Noble, A. (2018). Mental health disparities among college students of color. *Journal of Adolescent Health, 63*, 348–356. https://doi.org/10.1016/j.jadohealth.2018.04.014

Littrell, J., & Beck, E. (2001). Predictors of depression in a sample of African-American homeless men: Identifying effective coping strategies given varying levels of daily stressors. *Community Mental Health Journal, 37*(1), 15–29.

Locks, A.M, Hurtado, S., Bowman, N. A., Oseguera, L. (2008). Extending Notions of Campus Climate and Diversity to Students' Transition to College. *The Review of Higher Education, 31*(3), 257-285. Project MUSE, https://doi.org/10.1353/rhe.2008.0011.

Lundy-Wagner, V., & Gasman, M. (2011). When gender issues are not just about women: Reconsidering male students at historically black colleges and universities. *Teachers College Record, 113*(5), 934–968.

Martin, J. M. (2010). Stigma and student mental health in higher education. *Higher Education Research & Development, 29*(3), 259–274. https://doi.org/10.1080/07294360903470969

Masuda, A., & Boone, M. S. (2011). Mental health stigma, self-concealment, and help-seeking attitudes among Asian American and European American college students with no help-seeking experience. *International Journal for the Advancement of Counselling, 33*(4), 266–279. https://doi.org/10.1007/s10447-011-9129-1

McGowan, B. L. (2016). Interpersonal relationships: Exploring race and relationship decisions among African American college men. *Journal of Student Affairs Research and Practice, 53*(3), 243–255. https://doi.org/10.1080/19496591.2016.1118381

McGowan, B. L., & Pérez, D. (2020). A community built just for me: Black undergraduate men bridging gaps to community cultural wealth. *Journal of The First-Year Experience & Students in Transition, 32*(1), 43–57.

Mincey, K., Alfonso, M., Hackney, A., & Luque, J. (2014). Understanding masculinity in undergraduate African American men: A qualitative study. *American Journal of Men's Health, 8*(5), 387–398. https://doi.org/10.1177/1557988313515900

Morgan, C., & Cotton, S. R. (2003). The relationship between internet activities and depressive symptoms in a sample of college freshmen. *Cyberpsychology & Behavior, 6*(2), 133–142. https://doi.org/10.1089/109493103321640329

Mushonga, D. R., & Henneberger, A. K. (2020). Protective factors associated with positive mental health in traditional and nontraditional black students. *American Journal of Orthopsychiatry, 90*(1), 147–160. https://doi.org/10.1037/ort0000409

National Center for Education Statistics. (2020). Immediate college enrollment rate. The condition of education. https://nces.ed.gov/programs/coe/indicator_cpa.asp

Naumann, W. C., Bandalos, D., & Gutkin, T. B. (2003). Identifying variables that predict college success for first-generation college students. *Journal of College Admission, 181*, 4–9.

Oh, H. J., Ozkaya, E., & LaRose, R. (2014). How does online social networking enhance life satisfaction? The relationships among online supportive interaction, affect, perceived social support, sense of community, and life satisfaction. *Computers in Human Behavior, 30*, 69–78. https://doi.org/10.1016/j.chb.2013.07.053

Oliver, W. (2006). "The streets" an alternative black male socialization institution. *Journal of Black Studies, 36*(6), 918–937. https://doi.org/10.1177/0021934704273445

Oliver, M. D., Datta, S., & Baldwin, D. R. (2017). Wellness among African-American and Caucasian students attending a predominantly white institution. *Journal of Health Psychology, 24*(12), 1637–1645. https://doi.org/10.1177/1359105317694484

Owens, D., Lacey, K., Rawls, G., & Holbert-Quince, J. A. (2010). First-generation African American male college students: Implications for career counsellors. *The Career Development Quarterly, 58*(4), 291–300.

Palmer, R., & Gasman, M. (2008). "It takes a village to raise a child": The role of social capital in promoting academic success for African American men at a black college. *Journal of College Student Development, 49*(1), 52–70. https://doi.org/10.1353/csd.2008.0002

Palmer, R. T., Davis, R. J., & Hilton, A. A. (2009). Exploring challenges that threaten to impede the academic success of academically underprepared black males at an HBCU. *Journal of College Student Development, 50*(4), 429–445. https://doi.org/10.1353/csd.0.0078

Pascarella, E. T., Pierson, C. T., Wolniak, G. C., & Terenzini, P. T. (2004). First-generation college students: Additional evidence on college experiences and outcomes. *The Journal of Higher Education, 75*(3), 249–284. https://doi.org/10.1353/jhe.2004.0016

Patton, L. D., Bridges, B. K., & Flowers, L. A. (2011). Effects of Greek affiliation on African American students' engagement: Differences by college racial composition. *College Student Affairs Journal, 29*(2), 113–123.

Payne, Y. A. (2011). Site of resilience: A reconceptualization of resiliency and resilience in street life–oriented black men. *Journal of Black Psychology, 37*(4), 426–451. https://doi.org/10.1177/0095798410394178

Perry, M. J. (2009). Black women earning college degrees outnumber college-educated black men 2 to 1. American Enterprise Institute. https://www.aei.org/carpe-diem/black-women-earning-college-degrees-outnumber-college-educated-black-men-2-to-1/

Petty, T. (2014). Motivating first-generation students to academic success and college completion. *College Student Journal, 48*(1), 133–140.

Plowden, K. O., & Young, A. F. (2003). Sociostructural factors influencing health behaviors of urban African American men. *Journal of the National Black Nurses Assoc, 14*(1), 45–51.

Plowden, K. O., John, W., Vasquez, E., & Kimani, J. (2006). Reaching African American men: A qualitative analysis. *Journal of Community Health Nursing, 23*(3), 147–158. https://doi.org/10.1207/s15327655jchn2303_2

Próspero, M., Russell, A. C., & Vohra-Gupta, S. (2012). Effects of motivation on educational attainment: Ethnic and developmental differences among first-generation students. *Journal of Hispanic Higher Education, 11*(1), 100–119. https://doi.org/10.1177/1538192711435556

Rafal, G., Gatto, A., & DeBate, R. (2018). Mental health literacy, stigma, and help-seeking behaviours among male college students. *Journal of American College Health, 66*(4), 284–291. https://doi.org/10.1080/07448481.2018.1434780

Ratnayake, P., & Hyde, C. (2019). Mental health literacy, help-seeking behaviour and wellbeing in young people: Implications for practice. *The Educational and Developmental Psychologist, 36*(1), 16–21. https://doi.org/10.1017/edp.2019.1

Seifert, T. A., Drummond, J., & Pascarella, E. T. (2006). African-American students' experiences of good practices: A comparison of institutional type. *Journal of College Student Development, 47*(2), 185–205. https://doi.org/10.1353/csd.2006.0023

Seroalo, K. B., Du Plessis, E., Koen, M. P., & Koen, V. (2014). A critical synthesis of interventions to reduce stigma attached to mental illness. *Health SA Gesondheid, 19*(1), 80010. https://doi.org/10.4102/hsag.v19i1.800

Sharac, J., McCrone, P., Clement, S., & Thornicroft, G. (2010). The economic impact of mental health stigma and discrimination: A systematic review. *Epidemiology and Psychiatric Sciences, 19*(3), 223–232. https://doi.org/10.1017/s1121189x00001159

Soria, K. M., & Stebleton, M. J. (2012). First-generation students' academic engagement and retention. *Teaching in Higher Education, 17*(6), 673–685. https://doi.org/10.1080/1356251 7.2012.666735

Stephens, N. M., Fryberg, S. A., Markus, H. R., Johnson, C. S., & Covarrubias, R. (2012). Unseen disadvantage: How American universities' focus on independence undermines the academic performance of first-generation college students. *Journal of Personality and Social Psychology, 102*(6), 1178–1197. https://doi.org/10.1037/a0027143

Strand, K. J. (2013). *Making sure they make it! Best practices for ensuring the academic success of first-generation college students. CIC/Walmart college success awards report.* Council of Independent Colleges. https://files.eric.ed.gov/fulltext/ED561082.pdf

Strayhorn, T. L. (2008). The role of supportive relationships in facilitating African American males' success in college. *NASPA Journal, 45*(1), 26–48. https://doi.org/10.2202/1949-6605.1906

Taylor, S. Z. (2018). *African American and first-generation students' perceptions of and experiences with an academic cohort* (publication no. 1036). [doctoral dissertation, University of Mississippi]. Electronic theses and dissertations. https://egrove.olemiss.edu/etd/1036

Thayer, P. B. (2000). Retention of students from first generation and low-income backgrounds. In *Opportunity outlook: The journal of the Council for Opportunity in education. Short paper.* National TRI Clearing House.

Van Der Gaag, M., & Snijders, T. A. B. (2005). The resource generator: Social capital quantification with concrete items. *Social Networks, 27*(1), 1–29. https://doi.org/10.1016/j.socnet.2004.10.001

Vasquez-Salgado, Y., Greenfield, P. M., & Burgos-Cienfuegos, R. (2015). Exploring home-school value conflicts: Implications for academic achievement and Well-being among Latino first-generation college students. *Journal of Adolescent Research, 30*(3), 271–305. https://doi.org/10.1177/0743558414561297

Ward, L., Siegel, M. J., & Davenport, Z. (2012). *First-generation college students: Understanding and improving the experience from recruitment to commencement.* John Wiley & Sons.

Watkins, D. C. (2012). Depression over the adult life course for African American men: Toward a framework for research and practice. *American Journal of Men's Health, 6*(3), 194–210. https://doi.org/10.1177/1557988311424072

Watkins, D. C. (2019). Improving the living, learning, and thriving of young black men: A conceptual framework for reflection and projection. *International Journal of Environmental Research and Public Health, 16*, 1331. https://doi.org/10.3390/ijerph16081331

Watkins, D. C., & Jefferson, S. O. (2013). Recommendations for the use of online social support for African American men. *Psychological Services, 10*(3), 323–332. https://doi.org/10.1037/a0027904

Watkins, D. C., & Neighbors, H. W. (2007). An initial exploration of what 'mental health' means to young black men. *Journal of Men's Health and Gender, 4*(3), 271–282. https://doi.org/10.1016/j.jmhg.2007.06.006

Watkins, D. C., Green, B. L., Rivers, B. M., & Rowell, K. L. (2006). Depression and black men: Implications for future research. *Journal of Men's Health and Gender, 3*(3), 227–235.

Watkins, D. C., Green, B. L., Goodson, P., Guidry, J. J., & Stanley, C. A. (2007). Using focus groups to explore the stressful life events of black college men. *Journal of College Student Development, 48*(1), 105–118. https://doi.org/10.1353/csd.2007.0009

Watkins, D. C., Walker, R. L., & Griffith, D. M. (2010). A meta-study of black male mental health and Well-being. *Journal of Black Psychology, 36*(3), 303–330. https://doi.org/10.1177/0095798409353756

Watkins, D. C., Allen, J. O., Goodwill, J. R., & Noel, B. (2017). Strengths and weaknesses of the Young black men, masculinities, and mental health (YBMen) Facebook project. *American Journal of Orthopsychiatry, 87*(4), 392–401. https://doi.org/10.1037/ort0000229

Watkins, D. C., Goodwill, J. R., Johnson, N. C., Casanova, A., Wei, T., Allen, J. O., Williams, E. G., Anyiwo, N., Jackson, Z., Talley, L. M., & Abelson, J. M. (2020). An online behavioral health intervention promoting mental health, manhood, and social support for black men: The YBMen project. *American Journal of Men's Health, 14*(4), 1–17. https://doi.org/10.1177/1557988320937215

Womack, V. Y., & Sloan, L. R. (2017). The association of mindfulness and racial socialization messages on approach-oriented coping strategies among African Americans. *Journal of Black Studies, 48*(4), 408–426. https://doi.org/10.1177/0021934717696789

Wood, J. L., Hilton, A. A., & Lewis, C. (2011). Black male collegians in public two-year colleges: Student perspectives on the effect of employment on academic success. *National Association of Student Affairs Professionals Journal, 14*(1), 97–110.

Chapter 5
Situating for Success: Lessons Learned from the Evaluation of the Making Connections Place-based Mental Health Initiatives Involving Boys and Men of Colour Across the United States

Roxann McNeish Taormina, Ruben Cantu, and William Crary

Introduction: Background

Making Connections (MCI) is an initiative created to change community conditions that influence male mental health and wellbeing. Boys and men of colour (BMOC) were a primary focus of MCI. They are more likely to experience poor mental health and wellbeing due to multi-generational trauma, higher exposure to poverty, higher rates of incarceration, and other factors (see Prevention Institute, 2014 for a review). This population also faces barriers to early intervention, significant stigma associated with traditional mental health supports, and more frequent introduction of care through the criminal justice system. Peer-focused supports and community-based changes supporting prevention are challenging and most needed. Prevention requires changing community conditions to promote broader, healthier, and more inclusive perspectives on gender and ensuring gender-responsive support systems.

The initiative, which began in 2015, brought together 13 communities across the U.S. to shift policies, practices, and norms to create greater opportunities for mental health and resilience. The 13 sites in rural, urban, and suburban locations (four in the Western/Pacific region of the U.S., three in the Northeast, two in the South, two in the Southwest and two in the Central region) focused on improving social connections, economic and educational opportunities and assets, and the physical

R. M. Taormina (✉)
Department of Child and Family Studies, College of Behavioural and Community Sciences, University of South Florida, Tampa, FL, USA
e-mail: mcneish@usf.edu

R. Cantu · W. Crary
Prevention Institute, Oakland, CA, USA
e-mail: ruben@preventioninstitute.org; williamc@preventioninstitute.org

J. A. Smith et al. (eds.), *Health Promotion with Adolescent Boys and Young Men of Colour*, https://doi.org/10.1007/978-3-031-22174-3_5

73

environment. Activities varied by site, but included intergenerational mentor/men-tee programming, male-only peer groups, male-only drop-in centres, sports-based activities, training, community education, civic engagement activities, culture-based activities, gardening/caring for the land, and repairing bikes. Most sites focused on youth and young adult males, with the youngest participants being of elementary age (8 years old); two sites focused on adult males of colour. Participants were Black/African American, Hispanic, Native American/American Indian, Asian, and Pacific Islander males. The Making Connections Initiative (MCI) was funded by Movember, coordinated by Prevention Institute, and evaluated by a team at the University of South Florida.

MCI sites each included a primary grantee organisation and a collaborative of community organisations and members. Collaboratives developed strategies with their specific focus population and adopted gendered approaches for engagement and delivery. The collaboratives implemented community-level prevention strate-gies that reflected their communities' priorities, drawing on local or Indigenous knowledge, culture, and customs. Collaboratives also worked to deconstruct unhealthy norms around what it means to be a boy or man, and developed programs and policies that instilled healthier norms like social connection, civic engagement, and equitable relationships. Grantee organisations, which varied in size and scope, responded to the funding announcement, and directly received grant funds. In most cases, grantee staff were responsible for delivering programming directly, but others contracted with community partners to deliver programming while grantee staff provided oversight. All grantees were required to participate in the national cross-site evaluation, and some also had local evaluation support. In the latter case, the national evaluation team worked collaboratively with the local evaluators.

Background on the Evaluation

The MCI cross-site evaluation was primarily designed as an exploratory case study to enable site-specific assessment and cross-site comparisons. Qualitative data pro-vided an in-depth understanding of community and organisational contexts and implementation. Data sources included document review, monthly semi-structured grantee telephone interviews, and annual site visits that included observations as well as individual and/or group interviews with grantee staff, community partners, and participants. Quantitative data was collected using concept mapping and a community-informed outcome survey created for the MCI; partnerships were assessed using a standardized collaboration survey and network analysis.

Understanding that community change takes many years and was not likely to be fully realised over the five years of MCI, one goal of the evaluation was to assess the capacity of programs to create change and how this capacity was built during imple-mentation. Domains and related strategies that either strengthened or impeded grantee progress were identified from planning year (Year 1) data. Over the next four implementation years, data revealed that the domains remained constant, but strategies were added and revised when found to be facilitators or barriers to progress. The lessons learned, organised by domains and strategies, are discussed in this chapter.

Administrative Support

Administrative support includes structures and processes that facilitate day-to-day grant administration and project management. This can include, but is not limited to record-keeping; scheduling and facilitating meetings; communication, planning, and coordination of grant activities, including evaluation, staff training, and community engagement. Administrative support or facilitative administration (Bertram et al., 2015) is foundational to any initiative as it supports task identification, prioritization, execution, and delegation as needed.

An important lesson learned regarding both implementation and evaluation is the critical importance of clarity from funders and/or program administrators about program expectations. Program expectations should be clearly outlined at the beginning of the project and in all grantee documents/contracts. Evaluation needs and responsibilities should be made clear, particularly if there is an outside entity involved with the evaluation, but also so organisations can assess their internal evaluation capacity and make necessary decisions. These are particularly important considerations when working with communities of colour (CoC) as programs are often led by or involve smaller community-based organisations (Chaidez-Gutierrez & Fischer, 2013) and residents may exhibit mistrust of outside organisations (Park et al., 2018). Salient information such as data collection and reporting, as well as expectations regarding evaluation participation, should be made explicit. Data ownership and usage are other important issues that should be addressed early. Our findings, as well as the literature, highlight these as very important considerations when working with CoC (Hicks et al., 2012).

Lack of clarity about evaluation expectations contributed to many challenges for the cross-site evaluation team. These included: refusal to participate, limited participation, inconsistent participation, and wide variability in how and the extent to which local evaluations were conducted. Summarily, these challenges were addressed by building relationships with grant staff, their community partners, and program participants (when possible) while working collaboratively with the funder and program administrator to resolve these challenges iteratively.

On the other hand, we caution against being too prescriptive and rigid as to prevent communities from providing input into the program design and evaluation. Furthermore, the additional efforts invested in relationship and trust-building due to the lack of evaluation clarity increased opportunities for working collaboratively with grantee communities. The MCI evaluation included a technical assistance component, which enabled investing time in learning, teaching, and building. However, this investment would have been more challenging if the technical assistance role had been absent. Many community-based evaluations do not necessarily include this component or are done on an ad hoc basis. Our experience suggests that intentional investments in providing evaluation technical assistance benefits the community by building their capacity, and benefits the evaluation by creating opportunities to establish relationships with organizations and the community.

Organisational Leadership Involvement

The organisations involved in MCI that served BMOC varied in size and scope, and included public health and other large health organisations, midsize organisations, and small community-based grassroots organisations. A significant cross-site finding was that regardless of size, it was important that organisational leadership with decision-making capacity be involved in – or at least be aware of – the initiative. Leadership involvement helped prioritise MCI, address and dismantle administrative barriers in larger organisations (e.g., removing restrictive hiring requirements), and helped midsize and smaller organisations stay focused on MCI so it did not get lost or intertwined with their other initiatives. Research similarly indicates that executive-level involvement contributes to successful programs (Austin & Claiborne, 2011). Having leaders involved also helped bring awareness to the challenges that BMOC faced in many of these communities and helped increase leaders' recognition of the need and opportunities available to positively impact this population.

Staff Assignments and Commitment

Staff selection, training, and coaching are primary implementation drivers (National Implementation Research Network (NIRN, n.d.-a). Findings demonstrated the importance of having adequate staff assigned to MCI, having staff with the experience and/or training necessary to work with BMOC, and having staff committed to MCI's goals and the focus population. These factors affected all aspects of programming, including evaluation. Grantees that did not allocate sufficient staff time progressed slowly because many tasks, including evaluation, were either not completed or not completed well. Competing schedules or tasks within organisations can impede program activities and progression (Austin & Claiborne, 2011; Rieder et al., 2018). However, whether there was sufficient or limited staff, clarifying roles and clearly outlining responsibilities, particularly of the staff directly engaging with participants, facilitated implementation and evaluation.

Overall, staff needed a wide range of skills and experience to facilitate planning and implementation activities. Findings indicate that staff with program-planning experience enabled implementation to progress more than staff with content-area expertise (e.g., mental health) but no program-planning experience. These staff also progressed more than those who had experience conducting community programs but had limited program-planning experience. Staff with no prior experience work-ing with BMOC or CoC experienced more challenges initially engaging with par-ticipants and community organisations. Male staff of similar race/ethnicity and/or culture were more successful at engaging BMOC in programming compared to racially/ethically and culturally dissimilar males. Participants indicated that they were more comfortable with males they believed they could relate to and who could understand their experiences. Staff also needed to be observably committed to par-ticipants. Both BMOC participants and community partners acknowledged the importance of staff commitment in sustaining their engagement. Both stated that when the commitment was evident, they were more likely to overlook the lack of staff experience or shortcomings of the program and allow more time for improvement.

During implementation, it was important that there were opportunities to culti-vate and strengthen the skills of both staff and the focus population. Some MCI grantees provided opportunities for employment via grant funds or other programs (e.g., AmeriCorp). This was beneficial to the participants and often their families, the program, and the community as it promoted engagement, commitment, program sustainability, and created a future employment pathway. Mostly young males were provided these opportunities, and for some, it was their first 'official' position with an organisation. Training for grantee staff who predated MCI focused on increasing knowledge about beneficial interventions (e.g., restorative justice practices). At the same time, the young men were generally provided training on organisational prac-tices and working with participants in a leadership role. As an MCI goal was capac-ity building, training was also provided by the program administrator and evaluator on various program planning, implementation, and evaluation topics. The young leaders from different sites were also brought together throughout the initiative to share and learn from each other. This experience was reported to be one of the most valuable of MCI. One training need that would have benefitted the many young leaders and some staff was learning more about managing programs and the impor-tance of incorporating evaluation into program planning.

Evaluation Considerations

Leadership involvement also facilitated participation in the evaluation. When lead-ers were involved with program oversight, they generally were more likely to ensure that all aspects of the program were going well, including evaluation. They were also more likely to inquire about program impacts, prompting evaluation discussions.

Staff commitment also impacted participant engagement in evaluation. Staff who supported the evaluation, especially the cross-site evaluation, were more intentional and successful at data collection. Lack of staff commitment or support for the evalu-ation was a significant barrier. Staff were the conduit between the evaluation and program participants. When that connection was broken or not strong, it required grantee organisational leadership, the funder, and the program administrator to devise a solution. However, it is noteworthy that resistance was partly a result of the lack of clarity about evaluation expectations from the beginning of the project.

Involving all staff in evaluation extends and builds capacity of the program and the staff. It also facilitates program impact assessment by creating and seizing data collection opportunities. If only one or certain staff are involved in the evaluation, data collection opportunities are limited to their presence. This also does not convey the importance of evaluation as well as having all staff involved to some extent. Many grantees did not involve the BMOC leaders/staff in the evaluation, which proved to be an impactful missed opportunity.

Case Example: Administration Impacts Evaluation

This site focuses on Asian and Pacific Islander boys and young men. Primary engagement strategies included creating space for gathering, learning, and skill-building, civic engagement and community education, and leadership development. Their values encompassed authentic engagement with the community and focus population that was strengths-based and emphasised healing through storytelling and honouring place and identity. Like many community-based organisations, program staff were often focused on conducting activities that directly affected program participants. Evaluation was not always prioritised, not because of lack of ability, capacity, or any resistance, but because evaluation activities had not been incorporated into the overall program planning. Other contributing factors were lack of clarity about the local evaluation responsibilities and the importance of evaluation. The grantee organisation's leader, who had been less connected since the project began, had to be involved in the solution. An evaluator from the organisation was assigned to the MCI, and both the local and cross-site evaluations were prioritised moving forward. Including the local evaluator helped build the capacity of the project and the project staff due to having more meetings and discussions about evaluation.

Once evaluation expectations and importance were clarified, staff commitment to the evaluation increased. Staff were particularly important evaluation partners due to cultural practices and understandings at this site, which affected the evaluation. Being a story- and narrative-based culture, surveys were not the preferred means of assessment. MCI surveys had space for narrative responses, and on the first surveys participants completed, they skipped all the survey items and only answered the open-ended questions. Some participants provided paragraphs of written information. Participants did complete the survey items in subsequent administrations, as well as the open-ended questions because of staff working collaboratively with the evaluation team. Additionally, the survey language was standardised for use across sites and did not contain any colloquialisms, which they may have preferred. Having culturally responsive evaluations affirms the value of participants but often challenges funder expectations for quantifiable proof of impact. MCI provided some middle ground in that the cross-site evaluation was designed to capture program impact using mixed methods. Still, sites also had flexibility in the data they could collect as part of the local evaluation.

Leadership

Leadership is foundational to any program and program implementation. For the MCI evaluation, leadership was defined as a process by which an individual influences a group of individuals to achieve a common goal (Northouse, 2016). Defining leadership as an interactive process makes leadership open to many people rather than restricting leadership roles to individuals with formal leadership authority. Similarly, as an active implementation driver, leadership focuses on roles rather than just the position of a leader (NIRN, n.d.-b).

Many findings for leadership are similar to those for staff because, in many MCI communities, various staff held leadership roles. At all sites, a project director (P.D.) was responsible for grant oversight and management, and many had project coordinators (P.C.) responsible for programming. A few P.D.s were also involved in direct program delivery, but the P.C. (and other support staff) were often seen as the program lead by participants. Most BMOC sites were intentional about having a member of that population in a leadership role, which helped engagement. Boys and younger males were more likely to engage and remain engaged if project leaders were also men of colour. This was particularly important in the initial stages of implementation and engagement. The following factors related to leadership have also been found to support implementation.

Leadership Vision, Values, and Commitment

Leaders drive initiatives; their vision and commitment enable implementation to progress and continually move forward toward goals (Austin & Claiborne, 2011). Therefore, it is most beneficial when the leaders' vision aligns with the vision and expectations of the initiative. When this does not occur, findings indicate that project drift is very likely. This is a challenge for any program because it derails implementation and jeopardises the program's sustainability. When working with BMOC, this is always a risk because there are sometimes many needs and dedicated staff that want to serve in any way. Data show, however, that good intentions can sometimes lead to bad program planning. When leaders try to shape programs to their perception and be too responsive, this can diffuse activities to the point where there is minimal observable or documented impact. This is due to insufficient attention to these varied activities and not taking time to strategically design/choose and implement activities to reach program goals. Evaluation is adversely affected when this occurs.

Leadership Skills/Styles

A lot has been written about leadership and the types of leadership styles that are most effective. One framework, for example, outlines that technical and adaptive leadership helps initiate and manage needed change in organisations and systems (Active Implementation Research Network, n.d.). Similarly, findings from MCI showed that different leadership skills are needed to support implementation progress. Leaders who were both task-oriented and relationship-oriented were able to motivate partners and participants, problem solve, be open to input from others, as well as plan and remain focused on achieving outlined tasks. Task orientation (i.e., task-focused) was very effective in completing planned activities. However, in CoC, where trust and authenticity are important, building relationships and allowing others to provide input and share what they considered important to serving the community and BMOC was equally important.

Distributive/Shared Leadership

A strong facilitator to relationship building and implementation progress was having a distributive/shared leadership structure for MCI projects. Other benefits found for this type of leadership structure were increased commitment, sustained engagement, increased stability, and better management of impactful staff/leadership changes. This structure kept MCI staff accountable and enabled programs to adapt and remain relevant to the BMOC. Most youth-serving projects created youth advisory boards (YAB) to provide input into implementation activities, while others had BMOC as part of their MCI collaborative. Some sites created the YAB as part of the collaborative, but most kept it separate due to constraints on when board members could meet.

Leadership Development Opportunities

Providing leadership opportunities to BMOC was an important facilitator of implementation progress. Sites that provided leadership opportunities to young men had more sustained engagement. They were more committed to the program overall and were more likely to engage in other civic opportunities that positively impacted their community. Providing leadership opportunities appeared to ignite a desire and dedication to program success and sustainability. Having these opportunities provides tangible skills useful in many other areas, and provides a buffer against staff changes. Leadership opportunities also support positive youth development (Lin et al., 2018). One grantee allowed young men to become involved and have leadership responsibilities for the evaluation. This led to the increased commitment of the youth to getting participation in the evaluation, increased completion of program surveys, increased understanding of evaluation, and some youth becoming interested in learning more about evaluation outside of the grant.

Evaluation Considerations

Lack of leadership support for the evaluation was a major barrier. Staff interacting directly with participants were seen as leaders, regardless of their official title. They had more control over evaluation participation than the actual organizational grant leaders. Therefore, even if organizational leaders supported the evaluation, other grant leadership staff could hinder participation. This was experienced in the MCI. Therefore, it is crucial that all staff in leadership roles understand the importance of evaluation and commit to assisting in this process. Organizational grant leadership remains critical to evaluation as they will likely have to be involved in changing the behaviour and perceptions of other leaders.

Case Example: Leadership
This site focused on Black and Hispanic youth and young men. Activities focused on trauma-informed sports and play, mentoring, and building inter-generational connections. Elementary school boys were mentored by males 16 years or older. The leaders of this program have been integral to its successful implementation. Neither the P.D. nor the P.C. was familiar with community-based initiatives or working solely with BMOC. However, their commitment and dedication to the project were evident to the evaluation team and their partners from the very beginning. Partners reported that despite their inexperience, the leaders' enthusiasm and vision for the project ignited their enthusiasm. They also reported that these leaders were a primary reason they remained engaged with the project, amid implementation delays and other challenges. The leaders were task-focused but relational, recognising the importance of building relationships with partners they had never worked with or had worked with in a different capacity.

Though this site's leadership style was more centralized than distributive, this was done out of necessity rather than preference. Partners did not always have the time to provide input on activities when decisions needed to be made, but they tried to keep partners updated on activities in emails, newsletters, and meetings. Realising that clarifying tasks benefited partnership cohesion, there was a partner contract outlining roles and expectations based on partner input and preferences, which was modified yearly.

An important focus of the leaders was providing employment, training, and development opportunities to young men/mentors. They had to overcome many organisational barriers but ensured mentors were employees of the organization, not just contractors. They also addressed as many barriers as they could (e.g., transportation) and developed and delivered training to help mentors succeed in their leadership roles.

Partnership Development

Partners were defined as agencies and organisations participating in a community coalition to support the MCI vision and mission. All partnerships included at least one BMOC, agency representatives that served or were members of this population, or both. The following factors related to partnership development were found to support successful planning and implementation.

Building Trust

Trust had to be developed between the grantee organisation and partners, as well among partners. Partners described trust-building as developing through a considerable investment of time, sharing ideas, addressing preconceived notions of each other, and discussing perspectives on issues that affected the community. Many partners reported being surprised by the effort and the time needed for trust-building, but acknowledged that this was an integral process (McNeish et al., 2019). Some MCI partners worked together previously, which helped this process, but it was still necessary because no partners had worked together previously on this type of initiative. It took more time and effort for larger organisations to build trust. Most had not worked with partners in this type of collaborative and shared leadership capacity, or had not previously worked with BMOC or organisations that served this population. Importantly, these organisations had to acknowledge and address power differentials and create space for partners to participate in leadership and decision-making.

Purposeful Partnering

Partnering with organizations having a similar mission/vision to the MCI or committed to the population of focus was beneficial to initial and sustained planning and engagement of both partners and participants. These partners appeared more committed to the project and were more patient during challenges or implementation delays. However, if a partner's vision for the MCI or what was needed for BMOC did not align with the primary grantee's vision, the relationship became strained and usually discontinued. This occurred more often between larger organizations and grassroots community organizations.

Partnerships Can Expand Capacity

Partnering generally expanded the reach and capacity for impact of the MCI, similar to what has been found for other male mental health promotion programs in the literature (Robertson et al., 2018). Referred to as strategic partnering (McNeish et al., 2019), smaller community organisations would partner with larger organisations to bridge knowledge and resource gaps, while larger organisations partnered with smaller community organisations that had a more direct connection to the MCI communities and the trust of residents. Smaller community organisations, in particular, could increase their evaluation capacity by partnering with larger organisations or universities.

Partnering with Existing Community Leaders

Non-organisationally affiliated males were integral partners in the MCI in gaining the trust of community members. They were very beneficial in reaching and engaging participants, especially at sites focused on men or older youth. Many studies have highlighted the importance of community gatekeepers when working with CoC (Calva et al., 2020; Islam & Patel, 2018), and the MCI experience was no different. Males are generally less likely to get involved in programs (Rounds & Harvey, 2019; Stahlschmidt et al., 2013) so having men of colour community leaders involved in recruitment was beneficial to implementation progress. A lack of male program leaders has hindered recruitment (Gavarkovs et al., 2016).

Partnering with an Organisation

Usually, an organisational representative participates in a collaborative, and when that person leaves the organisation, the partner relationship is at risk. Since community organisations tend to have a fair amount of turnover, having a relationship with the partner organisation as a whole and not just its representative was most beneficial. If the leadership of the partner organisation is not aware of or committed to the initiative, that representative may not be replaced. Depending on that partner's role, this can create a gap and delay implementation.

A lack of role clarity can also delay implementation. Unclear roles, responsibilities, and expectations impeded implementation progress as it took more time to make decisions and complete tasks. Time is a limited commodity among partners who usually have many other responsibilities. When decision-making and task responsibilities were not clearly outlined, particularly in writing, this negatively affected partnership cohesion, which challenged partner engagement, commitment, and accountability.

Evaluation Considerations

Partners' involvement can expand evaluation capacity and activities, as well as accountability. Some MCI collaborative partners were responsible for specific grant activities. In these cases, data collection would have been easier as they had direct contact and often the trust of participants. Additionally, when partners held the project/staff accountable for implementation updates, including impact reports, it promoted evaluation activities. Unfortunately, there were missed opportunities in many MCI collaboratives, as they neither sufficiently informed or held partners accountable for evaluation responsibilities, nor did partners hold project staff accountable for reporting ongoing impact.

Case Example: Partnering

This site primarily focused on American Indian/ Native American elementary, middle, and high school students. Activities included implementing a school-based peer-to-peer curriculum to reduce suicide and promote Native mental health awareness in the community. The first P.D., a member of a tribe who was well known in the community, developed partnerships needed for the initial implementation stages. The next P.D. was an 'outsider' who joined the project when it was time to develop other partnerships to expand community outreach and get the program into schools. She benefited from the connections of the former P.D. and the reputation of the grantee organisation in the community, but had to take time to personally develop relationships and build trust with community organisations and members. This took time and the transition delayed implementation, but success would not have been possible without these partnerships.

Partners were strategically chosen based on what was needed to move activities forward. They were either members of organisations (e.g., the school district) or of the community and had connections that enabled access to the focus population. An integral partnership with a school district ended because of leadership changes in that organisation, but community connections and partners enabled the identification of a successful alternative. Partners are not always involved in day-to-day decision-making. Still, they have remained connected due to their commitment to the focus population and recognition of the need for this initiative.

This site had one of the most successful local and cross-site evaluations, largely due to their partnerships. Staff also always worked collaboratively with our cross-site evaluation team to ensure a comprehensive, non-duplicative, and responsive evaluation.

Community Engagement

Community engagement was defined as garnering the input, advice, and active participation of the community in the planning and implementation of the MCI. A community included both members-at-large, and members of the population of focus.

Other than the strategies already mentioned, sports-based programming was one of the most successful engagement strategies. Strategic communication plans that utilized male-friendly verbiage for social media and other communication platforms were helpful in engaging BMOC, as were genuine and authentic communication and interactions. Incentives were an effective strategy for increasing reach and attendance, but not for sustained engagement. Sites also consistently raised the importance of incorporating pillars of wellbeing, such as values of trust, belonging/ connection, safety, dignity, hope, and self-determination in programming, which they viewed as necessary for both individuals and communities to thrive. The following factors were found to support community engagement and implementation progress.

Building Trust

Trust-building is a pervasive theme when working with BMOC and community organisations that serve this population. This is paramount when considering engagement in CoC due to the mistrust that exists because of historical abuses and current perceptions of racism and discrimination. Trust-building was essential to implementation progress and was a primary facilitator to the successful engagement of BMOC. Initially, community members expressed concerns about participating in another program from which they might not receive much in return, providing information about themselves and not knowing or benefitting from the results, and having "outsiders" make decisions about community problems and solutions. Research has long indicated that CoC are often concerned about *just another program* collecting information, but not returning it (Lewis et al., 2002). MCI grantees tried to build trust in various ways, but the overarching strategy was involvement and inclusion. Involving community members in all aspects of programming, from beginning to end, was the most successful trust-building strategy.

Involving the Community Early

Needs assessment is usually the first step when planning to implement community programs. Involving the community in identifying needs and developing potential solutions increases commitment, as well as program relevance and impact.

Lefkowich et al. (2017) similarly found that involving participants in planning helps to promote program acceptability and accessibility. Involving members as participants and as project team members in community-facing roles benefits data collection and program design. Community members can help contextualise and clarify data, also helping to enhance partners' commitment to the program. MCI partners reported that participating in the needs assessment process helped increase their commitment to the initiative, as they could see and engage with those who would be directly impacted. Other programs also found that involvement in needs assessment resulted in increased interests and committed participation (Lewis et al., 2002).

Empowering the Population of Focus

Empowering BMOC to be agents in their own destiny and agents of change is a powerful tool to transform individuals and communities. Participants were engaged to varying extents in the different MCI communities, but data indicates that involvement begets engagement. Being involved in planning and other activities resulted in youth being empowered to participate and represent the MCI in the community, as well as engage in other community advocacy and civic efforts. This occurred even when no direct incentive was offered. Participant engagement also motivated community partners to support the initiative; partners were motivated by seeing the commitment and dedication of the participants.

Engaging with Community Members

MCI grantees were required to engage non-participant community members in some aspect of the project. One reason for doing this was to increase community male mental health awareness. The evaluation also involved surveying residents regarding their perception of the mental health of men and boys in the community. Most grantees reached the wider community by having annual or quarterly community events. These included mental health fairs, conferences, bike rides, community conversations, cultural events, food-based gatherings (e.g., dinners), and information tables at other community events. Incentives in the form of food, activities, or other logoed merchandise were an effective outreach tool.

Evaluation Considerations

Building trust in the evaluation and its processes is just as important as building trust for other aspects of programming. Involving staff, partners, and BMOC (when possible) in the evaluation processes facilitates trust-building. Remaining accessible and flexible throughout the process also promotes trust. There should be ongoing efforts to make the evaluation relevant and respectful of the community's history and culture. This benefits the evaluation by promoting involvement, but also benefits the community by capturing useful information. Sharing findings increases potential utility and improves relationships between community members and the evaluation team.

Case Example: Community Engagement

This site served East African boys and young men. Primary activities included a drop-in centre, community mental health conversations, various workshops, and sports. Engagement was initially successful due to partnerships, and the P.D. was both well-known in the community and a member of the focus population. They began with the drop-in centre, workshops, and gathering, but saw engagement dwindling after a while. Noticing that when participants gathered, they often played sports in a small area attached to the centre, staff and participants collaboratively decided that creating an organised sports program would be most beneficial to increase engagement. As a result, engagement increased about three-fold in a short period of time. This grantee always had some participants in leadership roles, though some roles did not become more formalised until participation increased. Youth leaders helped manage the influx of participants and helped keep the program responsive and relevant to their needs.

They also modelled the project's culture of openness and safety in efforts to destigmatize talking about mental health. This was very evident during community conversations; even with culturally sensitive topics, the young men were active in discussions. Participants were also active in other community efforts that benefited their community, such as protests and advocating for changes with local elected officials.

Staff worked collaboratively with the cross-site evaluation team, though it took them some time to plan and implement their local evaluation. The capacity was there, but this was a small organisation that had many programs occurring at the same time. Incorporating evaluation in planning was not always prioritised, but staff were responsive to suggestions about improvements.

Conclusion

Placed-based community mental health initiatives involving BMOC have the potential to impact the lives of community members in many positive ways. Positioning these programs for success is important to helping overcome challenges inherent in implementing these programs. Lessons learned from the longitudinal evaluation of various MCIs provide insights into facilitatory implementation and evaluation strategies. The importance of clarifying expectations pre- and during programming cannot be overstated, as this sets the foundation for how processes are undertaken. Clarity of staff and partner roles is also important to implementation progress and evaluation as it supports trust-building. Building trust with CoC and BMOC is necessary for any implementation effort. Involvement in program planning and decision-making promotes trust, engagement, and commitment. Staff and other BMOC leaders increase engagement, as does providing physical activities. Organizations developing these initiatives should be intentional about having, partnering, or developing the capacity to administer and lead. Organizational capacity undergirds the program's capacity to achieve and document impact.

Sites that demonstrated strength and sufficient capacity in each of the domains outlined above were better able to sustain programming via continued funding. Lessons learned indicated that even if sites were strong in some areas, but weak in others, this challenged their ability to sustain. The domains are integrated and somewhat compensatory, but some capacity was needed in all areas for implementation progress and sustainability.

References

Active Implementation Research Network. (n.d.). *Implementation drivers*. Active Implementation Research Network. https://www.activeimplementation.org/frameworks/implementation-drivers/

Austin, S. A., & Claiborne, N. (2011). Faith wellness collaboration: A community-based approach to address type II diabetes disparities in an African-American community. *Social Work in Health Care, 50*(5), 360–375. https://doi.org/10.1080/00981389.2011.567128

Bertram, R. M., Blase, K. A., & Fixsen, D. L. (2015). Improving programs and outcomes implementation frameworks and organization change. *Research on Social Work Practice, 25*(4), 477–487. https://doi.org/10.1177/1049731514537687

Calva, A., Matthew, R. A., & Orpinas, P. (2020). Overcoming barriers: Practical strategies to assess Latinos living in low-income communities. *Health Promotion Practice, 21*(3), 355–362. https://doi.org/10.1177/1524839919837975

Chaidez-Gutierrez, F., & Fischer, R. L. (2013). Reflecting on grantee evaluation accountability to funders: Exploring power dynamics with grassroots organizations in communities of color. *Journal of Community Practice, 21*(4), 304–326. https://doi.org/10.1080/10705422.2013.846286

Gavarkovs, A. G., Burke, S. M., Reilly, K. C., & Petrella, R. J. (2016). Barriers to recruiting men into chronic disease prevention and management programs in rural areas: Perspectives of program delivery staff. *American Journal of Men's Health, 10*(6), NP155–NP157. https://doi.org/10.1177/1557988315596226

Hicks, S., Duran, B., Wallerstein, N., Avila, M., Belone, L., Lucero, J., Magarati, M., Mainer, E., Martin, D., Muhammad, M., Oetzel, J., Pearson, C., Sahota, P., Simonds, V., Sussman, A., Tafoya, G., & Hat, E. W. (2012). Evaluating community-based participatory research to improve community-partnered science and community health. *Program in Community Health Partnerships: Research, Education, and Action, 6*(3), 289–299. https://doi.org/10.1353/cpr.2012.0049

Islam, N., & Patel, S. (2018). Best practices for partnering with ethnic minority-serving religious organizations on health promotion and prevention. *AMA Journal of Ethics, 20*(7), E643–E654. https://doi.org/10.1001/amajethics.2018.643

Lefkowich, M., Richardson, N., & Robertson, S. (2017). "If we want to get men in, then we need to ask men what they want": Pathways to effective health programming for men. *American Journal of Men's Health, 11*(5), 1512–1524. https://doi.org/10.1177/1557988315617825

Lin, J. L. L., Chan, M., Kwong, K., & Au, L. (2018). Promoting positive youth development for Asian American youth in a Teen Resource Center: Key components, outcomes, and lessons learned. *Children and Youth Services Review, 91*, 413–423. https://doi.org/10.1016/j.childyouth.2018.06.040

McNeish, R., Rigg, K. K., Tran, Q., & Hodges, S. (2019). Community-based behavioral health interventions: Developing strong community partnerships. *Evaluation and Program Planning, 73*, 111–115. https://doi.org/10.1016/j.evalprogplan.2018.12.005

National Implementation Research Network. (n.d.-a). *Framework 3: Implementation drivers*. National Implementation Research Network. https://nirn.fpg.unc.edu/module-1/implementation-drivers

National Implementation Research Network. (n.d.-b). *Leadership*. National Implementation Research Network. https://nirn.fpg.unc.edu/module-1/implementation-drivers/leadership-drivers

Northouse, P. G. (2016). *Leadership: Theory and Practice*. Sage Publications

Park, S., Mosley, J. E., & Grogan, C. M. (2018). Do residents of low-income communities trust organizations to speak on their behalf? Differences by organizational type. *Urban Affairs Review, 54*(1), 137–164. https://doi.org/10.1177/1078087416669059

Prevention Institute. (2014). *Making connections for mental health and wellbeing among men and boys in the U.S.: A report on the mental health and wellbeing of men and boys in the U.S. and opportunities to advance outcomes related to prevention, early intervention and stigma reduction*. Prevention Institute. https://www.preventioninstitute.org/publications/making-connections-mental-health-and-wellbeing-among-men-and-boys-us

Rieder, J., Cain, A., Carson, E., Benya, A., Meissner, P., Isasi, C. R., Wylie-Rosett, J., Hoffman, N., Kelly, C., Silver, E. J., & Bauman, L. J. (2018). Pilot project to integrate community and clinical level systems to address health disparities in preventing and treating obesity among ethnic minority inner-city middle school students: Lessons learned. *Journal of Obesity, 2018*, 6983936. https://doi.org/10.1155/2018/6983936

Robertson, S., Gough, B., Hanna, E., Raine, G., Robinson, M., Seims, A., & White, A. (2018). Successful mental health promotion with men: The evidence from 'tacit knowledge'. *Health Promotion International, 33*(2), 334–344. https://doi.org/10.1093/heapro/daw067

Rounds, T., & Harvey, J. (2019). Enrollment challenges: Recruiting men to weight loss interventions. *American Journal of Men's Health, 13*(1), 1–7. https://doi.org/10.1177/1557988319832120

Stahlschmidt, M. J., Threlfall, J., Seay, K. D., Lewis, E. M., & Kohl, P. (2013). Recruiting fathers to parenting programs: Advice from dads and fatherhood program providers. *Children and Youth Services Review, 35*(10), 1734–1741. https://doi.org/10.1016/j.childyouth.2013.07.004

Chapter 6
"Where Are Our Men?": How the DUDES Club Has Supported Indigenous Men in British Columbia, Canada to Seek a Path of Healing and Wellness

Paul A. Gross, Iloradanon H. Efimoff, Viviane Josewski, Frank Cohn, Sandy Lambert, Teka Everstz, and John Oliffe

Introduction

Indigenous Peoples of Canada have long suffered the consequences of colonization, much like other Indigenous Peoples around the world. The Canadian context in this regard is characterized in large part by the legacy of the Residential School System, which spanned from 1828 to 1997 (Truth and Reconciliation Commission of Canada [TRC], 2015a). This system was overseen by the Canadian government, in partnership with many churches in Canada at the time, via the Indian Act of 1876. The aim of the schools was to forcibly remove Indigenous children from their homes to be stripped of their language and culture while educated in mostly church-run schools

P. A. Gross (✉)
Department of Family Practice, University of British Columbia, Vancouver, BC, Canada

The Dudes Club, Vancouver, BC, Canada
e-mail: paul@dudesclub.ca

I. H. Efimoff
Department of Psychology, University of Manitoba, Winnipeg, MB, Canada
e-mail: efimoffi@myumanitoba.ca

V. Josewski
Faculty of Medicine, University of British Columbia, Okanagan, BC, Canada
e-mail: viviane.josewski@ubc.ca

F. Cohn · S. Lambert · T. Everstz
The Dudes Club, Vancouver, BC, Canada
e-mail: frank@dudesclub.ca; sandy@dudesclub.ca; teka@dudesclub.ca

J. Oliffe
Men's Health Research Program, School of Nursing, University of British Columbia, Vancouver, BC, Canada
e-mail: john.oliffe@ubc.ca

© The Editor(s) (if applicable) and The Author(s), under exclusive license to Springer Nature Switzerland AG 2023
J. A. Smith et al. (eds.), *Health Promotion with Adolescent Boys and Young Men of Colour*, https://doi.org/10.1007/978-3-031-22174-3_6

(TRC, 2015a). Thousands of children died at these schools (TRC, 2015a). The ongoing intergenerational traumas that have resulted from this system and many other ongoing racist, destructive government policies (e.g., the "Sixties Scoop," when thousands of Indigenous children were removed from homes deemed unsafe by social services) has sadly led to numerous poor health and social outcomes for Indigenous Peoples of Canada (Adelson, 2005; Allan & Smylie, 2015; Greenwood et al., 2015).

To document the toll of Residential Schools and guide and inspire reconciliation in Canada, the TRC was carried out from 2008 to 2015. As a result of this extensive work, the TRC published 94 Calls to Action to "redress the legacy of residential schools and advance the process of Canadian reconciliation" (TRC, 2015b). Many organizations in Canada attempt to address these Calls to Action, either led by or in partnership with Indigenous people and their communities. However, very few of these organizations focus on the health and wellbeing of Indigenous boys and men.

One such organization is the DUDES Club, which began in 2010 in Vancouver's Downtown Eastside (DTES) at the Vancouver Native Health Society, a local health clinic and drop-in centre (Efimoff et al., 2021; Gross et al., 2016). The DTES is one of Canada's most marginalized communities with exceptionally high rates of home-lessness, poverty, substance overuse, crime, and poor health outcomes (Krausz & Jang, 2015). These conditions have all been dramatically amplified by the opioid crisis in the last five years where First Nations people[1] across British Columbia were five times more likely than the general population to experience an overdose and three times more likely to die of an overdose (First Nations Health Authority [FNHA], 2017). In addition, 82% of all overdose deaths in 2018 were men (regard-less of ethnicity) (Henry, 2018). The DUDES Club is a participant-led initiative to support men in building healthy relationships, engaging in healthcare (Efimoff et al., 2021), and promoting Indigenous health and wellness worldviews (Gross et al., 2016). Each DUDES Club aims to provide a sanctuary where men can "take off their armour" and be open about any physical, mental, emotional, or spiritual challenges they may be facing. DUDES Clubs are run by local men who plan and coordinate the activities that help break the cycle of silence and isolation that all too often contribute to poor health and social outcomes for men (Goldenberg, 2014). DUDES Clubs facilitate a space where men can enhance their connection to com-munity, oneself, Indigenous language, culture, and Mother Nature (through land-based activities like ice-fishing, going out on trap lines, seasonal harvesting, and retreats). We believe that a meaningful connection to these elements is vital to good health and wellness. In addition, DUDES Clubs are founded on values of non-judgment and inclusion, creating a welcoming environment for all members who identify as men (Efimoff et al., 2021). Conversations about the impact of gender on health and wellness are frequent at DUDES Club gatherings. Local leaders and DUDES Club staff often apply evolving and deconstructing concepts of masculinity in carrying out their work. Since its inception, the DUDES Club has supported 50 sites throughout British Columbia (Fig. 6.1), most of which are located in Indigenous communities in the northern part of the province thanks to a successful partnership with the First Nations Health Authority (FNHA). The DUDES Club Society

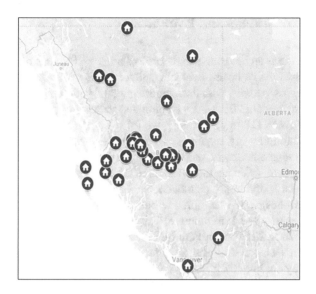

Fig. 6.1 Map of British Columbia with all DUDES Club sites. (DUDES Club, n.d.a)

officially became a registered Society and Charitable Organization in March 2020, working in partnership with many academic, governmental, non-profit, and community-level organizations.

The DUDES Club has demonstrated a sustainable, meaningful, and consistent impact across its sites over the years. We conducted extensive research and evaluation in 2013–2016 (thanks to funding from the Movember Foundation) and again in 2020 (thanks to a partnership between the Canadian Men's Health Foundation and FNHA). These efforts were always community-driven and designed with the support of DUDES Club team staff along with academic and governmental colleagues. From the very beginning, the intention was to follow a grassroots "organic" growth model in which participants determined which outcomes were most meaningful to them and their communities. As one participant so eloquently stated: "We once had this discussion about management executive decisions, they don't make them, this is by us, about us, and for us" (DUDES Club, 2021). As such, the impacts measured by the research and evaluation have intentionally been directly relevant to the men.

Furthermore, capturing the powerful narratives of DUDES Club members has been a central focus of our evaluation work. Throughout this chapter, we tell the story of the DUDES Club using a mixed-methods approach while honouring the lived experiences of the men who have contributed to, and benefited from, this movement for men's health and wellness in British Columbia, Canada. We also emphasize the importance of the intergenerational impacts and our work with adolescent and young men who direct innovative programs of their own (i.e., NexUp) inspired by the DUDES Club model. Finally, it is with a deep appreciation for, and respect of the traditions and worldviews of the many Indigenous Peoples of British Columbia that we share the story of the DUDES Club with you.

Quantitative Findings and Evaluation

The DUDES Club is an innovative and decolonising[1 model for] men's health promotion that destigmatises men's health issues by supporting men in accessing health care services on their own terms, with the support and affirmation of other men (Efimoff et al., 2021; Gross et al., 2016). As we continued to develop the DUDES Club program in Vancouver's DTES community, we received more interest from academic colleagues and funding organizations. To demonstrate the impact of the DUDES Club and encourage other communities to adopt a similar model in their setting, we were encouraged to evaluate the DUDES Club model. The leadership team of DUDES Club (i.e., community members, medical and social service providers, and academic colleagues) were committed to pursuing evaluation methods that aligned with the participatory and community-driven nature of the DUDES Club. The ideal opportunity came in 2013 when, with funding from the Movember Foundation, we joined the Men's Depression and Suicide Network at the University of British Columbia, led by Dr. John Oliffe and Dr. John Ogrodniczuk. The three-year research program was designed to engage five different projects highlighting innovative approaches to promoting men's mental health in Canada.

We contributed to this network with a program evaluation of the Vancouver DUDES Club and an iterative scale-up of three DUDES Club pilot sites in diverse community settings in Northern British Columbia. The evaluation was designed with the support of a community advisory committee composed of Elders, DUDES Club members, academics, and service providers. In our mixed-methods approach, we used both a quantitative survey and qualitative focus groups and individual interviews. The survey was developed using an applied logic model approach grounded in Indigenous wellness perspectives (i.e., medicine wheel teachings of balance between mental, physical, emotional, and spiritual dimensions of health). We administered the evaluation survey to 150 men at the Vancouver DUDES Club from 2014–2015 (Gross et al., 2016). In the article by Gross et al. (2016), readers can find a detailed description of the history and function of the Vancouver DUDES Club in its early years when an innovative blend of safety, comfort, support services, food, and cultural teachings empowered men to connect and improve their overall health and wellbeing.

There were two main findings in the evaluation survey. The first was a positive correlation between frequency of attendance and a greater overall benefit across the four dimensions of the medicine wheel (Fig. 6.2). This "dose-response" relationship was of value and also encouraging as it indicated that consistent attendance was related to better health and wellness outcomes. Furthermore, this finding emphasized the essential power of a space that prioritizes consistent relationships between the participants, leaders, and professional service providers. This relational practice has gradually become the cornerstone of DUDES Club and is one of the core values of our work. The second salient finding from the evaluation survey was that DUDES Club members who identify as Indigenous reported a greater sense of trust, social support, and improved connection to their cultural heritage when compared to

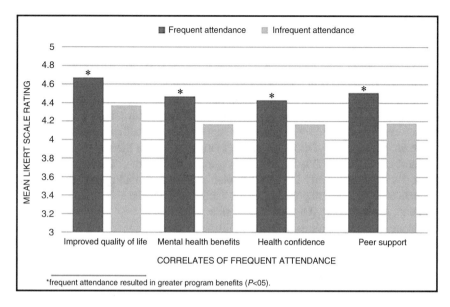

Fig. 6.2 Frequent Attendance Improves Outcomes. (Gross et al., 2016)

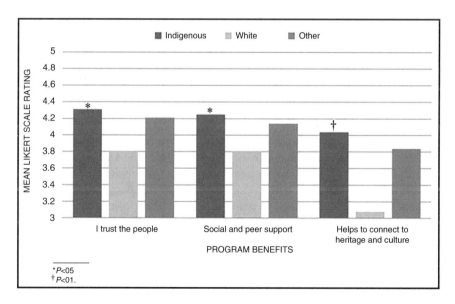

Fig. 6.3 Outcomes by Ethnic Identification. (Gross et al., 2016)

members who did not identify as Indigenous (Fig. 6.3). This was strong evidence that the DUDES Club is a culturally safe space where Indigenous men could reclaim aspects of their identity that had been stolen as a result of colonisation.

Recent publications further reinforce the impact of the DUDES Club and similar models for marginalized populations affected by social and health inequities, such as Indigenous boys and men, around the world. For example, the importance of health literacy, particularly for isolated men experiencing poverty and low education, has been highlighted as a consideration for effective program design in Canada (Oliffe, McCreary, et al., 2020a). In Australia, Smith et al. (2019) demonstrated the importance of addressing similar social determinants of health like employment, housing, education, youth incarceration, and the importance of social support in relation to the health of young Aboriginal and Torres Strait Islander males. Open and informative health discussions, often supported by a health professional or local Elder, are central to DUDES Club and help improve health literacy for all involved (Efimoff et al., 2021). This is just one example of a variety of important considerations for designing men's health promotion programs including ongoing program evaluation and a focus on populations most affected by social and structural marginalization, among others (Oliffe, Rossnagel, et al., 2020b).

The quantitative findings from the evaluation survey (Gross et al., 2016) laid the foundation for our continual process of grassroots, organic and iterative program design. This process provides a fertile environment for men to cultivate individual and collective agency through their engagement in the DUDES Club. For instance, men are encouraged to move along a trajectory from being silent or avoidant about their health and social connections to becoming curious and interested, and ultimately, to serious and committed. This impact, among many others, is described in richer detail through the qualitative observations of the Movember-funded evaluation (Efimoff et al., 2021), summarized in the following section of this chapter.

In 2016 the First Nations Health Authority (FNHA) Northern Region began an extensive and ongoing collaboration with the DUDES Club Society (DCS) to respond to the need of addressing men's health in more direct ways. This was initiated during the planning for the first Northern Guys Gathering in 2017, followed by a series of community support visits, consultations on hiring a Northern Men's Wellness Coordinator, land-based retreats, and 10 sub-regional Train-the-Trainer events for Elders and facilitators from more than 35 northern communities. These activities led to the development of Indigenous Men's wellness groups meeting regularly, involving 32 of the 54 northern First Nations communities. That changed with the COVID-19 Pandemic when communities had to make adjustments, taking their activities online, outdoors, or going on hiatus. These community sites have benefited from the innovative public-private partnership with the FNHA (Northern Region) that provides the groups with a modest amount of annual funding ($7500) allocated to meals, traditional activities (e.g., drum-making, canoeing, singing), or other wellness activities (e.g., nature walks, talking circles) decided upon by the local group.

In 2020, having reached our fourth year of collaboration with FNHA Northern Region, we conducted a survey-based evaluation (for the full report referenced in this section, see DUDES Club, n.d.b). To create this survey, we started with our original evaluation survey (see Gross et al., 2016) and refined the questions through a series of advisory consultations with the DUDES Club members, community leadership, and FNHA staff. We had 139 participants respond from 23 communities. Most respondents (99) were living on-reserve, with the rest (40) in urban centres.

The urban sites show diversity with an increased number of men away from their home territories and traditional teachings, and also an increased number of men who did not identify as being Indigenous. With few exceptions, community (on-reserve) sites tended to be composed entirely of Indigenous men. In contrast, approximately 65–70% of DUDES members at urban sites are Indigenous (membership at the urban DUDES Club sites is more transient making accurate attendance data difficult; this approximation is based on discussions with our urban site coordinators and leaders). Importantly, when comparing Indigenous and non-Indigenous men, the results of both the 2020 and 2013–2016 surveys indicated that Indigenous respondents consistently expressed higher levels of satisfaction with DUDES Club.

For our 2020 survey, we used two very similar surveys: one questionnaire for urban sites and one for community sites. Both surveys included survey questions covering health services, connection to culture, relationships with others, and overall satisfaction with the program. Respondents in the survey cited significant benefits from participating in their respective DUDES Clubs, including social and peer support, connection to heritage and culture, trust in other people, community participation, and awareness of healthcare services. Highlights of the survey data include the following:

- 96.38% of respondents would recommend the DUDES Club to other men
- 84.00% reported an increased awareness of health services
- 85.56% reported that their health had improved
- 82.83% reported an increase in the use of their voice
- 82.8% reported increased community participation
- 84.10% reported an increase in trusting others

The men we work with have consistently told us that, pre-colonization, they would come together in community. Colonization has disrupted the traditional ways in which men would gather. DUDES Club is helping to change that. According to a DUDES Club facilitator in the community of McLeod Lake in North Central BC: "Men are building men's confidence. Men are having pride in themselves. It has helped change the dynamics of the reserve." In the island village of Gitxaala on B.C.'s Central Coast, the facilitator has seen "an increase in pride in the community and an increase in community unity." He adds that the community drug and alcohol counsellor attends gatherings as a support for the DUDES Club and is welcomed in that setting. "Guys in the Gitxaala club have developed ideas for projects that are sparking motivation in other men."

Qualitative Findings

"We look after each other as DUDES, we're a brotherhood of men."

In this section, we draw from our thematic analysis of 15 focus groups with approximately 100 DUDES Club members, Elders, and providers (Efimoff et al., 2021).

The rich qualitative findings we present here highlight four interwoven themes within men's narratives of being a DUDES Club member: (1) creating safe and inclusive spaces for men; (2) forging new connections and intergenerational relations; (3) reclaiming what it means to be a man and (4) decolonising healthcare.

Most men who attend the DUDES Club live with past and/or current experiences of trauma, violence, poverty, mental illness, and addictions issues as well as other stigmatized health conditions. These experiences spurred the men's need for safe spaces where they can "leave their armour at the door." Though men talked about valuing different aspects of the DUDES Club, most agreed that what made them want to come back to the DUDES Club was that it offered a space where "once you walk through that door you know you're safe." This sense of safety enabled men to form friendships with one another that contributed to a feeling of brotherhood and camaraderie among the members, and ultimately "a sense of belonging and community." As one man who frequently attended one of the DUDES Clubs explained:

> I think with the DUDES, our self-identity is really important and I think that's what many of us are looking for – like, how do I fit in … is there somebody that is going to accept me … and when you come into a DUDES meeting, there it is. You're not judged, you're able to speak in the way you wish, the way you're comfortable with, um, in a polite and respectful manner, whereas outside you may have to come across a little bit more gruff … that sort of thing.

As this man's narrative illustrates, men's everyday "armour" can be taken off. In many support-group and health-care settings, people may be turned away if they are actively using drugs. A key way the DUDES Club creates safety is by cultivating a non-judgmental and inclusive atmosphere where everyone, including those who are actively using drugs, are treated with respect and welcomed with dignity rather than turned away, as often happens in other support groups and settings, including health care. As one man commented:

> You can come in here and even if you are using drugs you talk about all kinds of stuff, it's nonjudgmental. That's the big thing, because you walk into most places and I'm an addict and this is a problem … I am just a fucking addict.

In several DUDES Clubs, members fostered respect and unconditional positive regard through the co-creation of rules of engagement that governed their interactions with one another. DUDES Clubs also used peer-based and peer-driven activities to promote self-care and caring for others among the men, such as free haircuts, fishing, tai chi, or serving food. Instead of sitting in a hierarchically-structured doctor's office to meet for a few minutes, members decide amongst themselves how they can best support one another as a community, and invite health providers to support where desired. This environment, where a community of men decide how to engage with and support one another, is arguably a way to decolonize health care interactions. DUDES Club members provided many examples of how simple acts of kindness and caring – such as giving and receiving a haircut – enhanced their sense of wellbeing and positive outlook. For example, one member said the free haircuts were "worth a million bucks" when talking about how they made the men feel. One man who self-identified as Indigenous reflected on his experiences of offering free haircuts to men during the DUDES Club meetings:

> [C]oming to this group and participating and volunteering … it also increases my aware-ness of what the guys are going through as well as [what] I'm going through….So you can communicate with one another especially when I'm cutting their hair… and … when a person gets their hair cut that also increases their confidence, their kindness, you know, like … it makes you feel good to walk out the door. … Guys … need to feel clean and keep grooming yourself, you know, like because sometimes after a while living down here, you basically give up.

For many men, the DUDES Club was identified as instrumental to their wellbeing, and often the only source of support in their lives. Repeatedly giving and receiving support from other men who share similar lived experiences was particularly power-ful, because it fostered an environment where men felt "able to trust … and open up a lot more" about their personal struggles and issues that mattered to them. Members discussed topics that are often considered controversial or taboo, such as substance use, depression, experiences of sexual abuse, and grief. In the voice of one man who had experienced the tragic loss of his son: "In a lot of ways it's saved me too, like, from depression, and at the time I was grieving, so in a lot of ways I returned to life ... Only men understand men and what they go through." Though healthcare provid-ers are often present at DUDES Club meetings to share health information with the men, consistent with a decolonising model of health care, the DUDES Club mem-bers decide what health issues they want to discuss and where the discussions go. As many of the men emphasized, the experience of "finally being heard and ... able to voice their concerns over things that are really bothering them" was profoundly meaningful. This was especially the case because of many members' experiences with healthcare providers outside the DUDES Club, as described by one participant: "they think they know all the answers … they think they can tell you what's wrong with you" and "they don't listen to what your real problems are."

Two issues that were at the forefront of many of the men's discussions were intergenerational engagement and being a father. For example, many members expressed the desire to mentor younger men, noting that "there's a lot of young men out there that are angry ... they've got nowhere to go, no one to talk to." One member saw the potential for DUDES Club members to be father figures while others dis-cussed the desire to pass on skills to the next generation of men. Perhaps not surpris-ingly, men valued being able to bring their children or grandchildren to the DUDES Club as "mini-DUDES" and having access to a safe space for discussing issues of fatherhood. This enabled them to challenge dominant masculine stereotypes and gender norms while reframing healthier strength-based ideals of masculinity. For example, one member described how the DUDES Club is helping men to get "to the point where they can be loving fathers and strong warriors ... at the same time." Contrary to the dominant ideals of masculinity, this man believed that "the two don't have to be exclusive." Such an open discussion of fatherhood pushes against the stereotypes that men are not nurturers and the male ideal of always needing to show up as the "strong and silent type." As one man shared, "you gotta cry, man.

You gotta. You can't hold it in." In addition, at one of the Northern B.C. communities, adolescent men would bring their sometimes-reluctant fathers and uncles along to DUDES Club meetings. This was a great example of how the intergenerational impact of the DUDES Club model is bidirectional and, depending on the context, can be designed to encourage the participation of younger and/or older men based on the preference in each community.

Many members also discussed ways to improve their DUDES Club's reach and to help the community. For example, one member discussed how he joined the DUDES Club to try to make the community safer for his children, saying "... I mean I want it to be safe for my children and I don't feel it's safe for them right now. So, I have to make a change. And that's why I joined the DUDES club." Members discussed how attending the DUDES Club not only improved their own wellness, but also improved their relationships with their partners, children, and the broader community, explaining that "the healthier the men in the community are, the healthier the whole community is." One healthcare provider described how a man returned to the DUDES Club to "thank" the members for providing him with the emotional support he needed to cope with a conflict in his relationship rather than getting "drunk," to use his words, as he said he would have done previously.

Other important sources of healing, resilience, and support that men – regardless of their ethnicity, but particularly Indigenous men – identified included (re)connecting with Indigenous culture and Elders. Elder Henry Charles, one of six fluent Musqueam speakers, encouraged all members to reconnect with their culture and relearn their language. Many participants acknowledged Elder Henry Charles's important role. One participant, for example, said "his stories, his smudges, and giving us an opportunity just to have something different. Maintain the culture." Participants also indicated they valued elders sharing their language:

> P1: I think it's great that he actually speaks in his own tongue.
> P2: And shares it with us.
> P3: Yeah, and shares it with us very openly, and that's very rare down here. Like, he's the only one that I think that I've ever actually heard speak his own language...
> P4: I speak my own language... [the elder's language is] a different dialect than my Chilcotin but I enjoy hearing it like, yeah. Some words I recognise...
> Elder Henry Charles carried and shared this knowledge with DUDES Club members until he joined the spirit world in 2017.

Although the role of Elders varied between DUDES Clubs, depending in part on the Elder's knowledge and their availability, there was a deep appreciation of having an Elder present. According to King and Gracey (2009), in many Indigenous cultures, "Elders are those who have shown wisdom and leadership in cultural, spiritual and historical matters within their communities, and might not necessarily be old. Elders represent an essential connection with the past; they are keepers of the community knowledge and supporters of its collective spirit" (p. 82). As described above, at one DUDES Club located in the inner city of a large metropolitan area, men described how the Indigenous Elder played a central role in reconnecting members to their cultural identity by sharing "traditional knowledge." This was especially significant given that disconnection from community and/or culture was common among the men due to such factors as geographic barriers, the legacy of colonial policies such as residential schooling, the Sixties Scoop, and current child welfare practices, and because cultural and language revitalization are increasingly recognized as important health promotion strategies for Indigenous Peoples (King & Gracey, 2009).

Future Directions

In the 2020 survey, we found that only 24.4% of respondents were under 40. Overall, this finding was consistent with the data from our earlier study which showed an average participant age of 46. In light of these findings, the DCS worked on developing new programs, namely NexUp, to attract younger participants to reduce social isolation and improve wellness among vulnerable populations of Indigenous youth and young men in B.C. We have yet to evaluate NexUp and briefly introduce this new and exciting initiative here.

The NexUp Initiative was launched in 2020 by DUDES Club staff members Ryan Avola and Teka Everstz. The goal is to build supportive and responsive strategies for the dynamic needs of the new youth and young adults. Nexup is a youth-focused, youth-built, and youth-led approach to health and wellness dedicated to building spaces that embrace Indigenous ways of knowing to support the spiritual, mental, emotional, and physical health of young men. Through collaborative community-based projects and activities, NexUp continues to uphold, enhance, support and advance the DCS mission and vision. NexUp works within communities with significant Indigenous populations, including urban neighbourhoods, small towns, rural villages, and on-reserve communities. NexUp focuses on supporting younger individuals during their unique learning journeys and encouraging continual collaboration on projects that focus on reimagining and redefining "men's health," as inspired by the DUDES Club model. An important part of re-imagining relationships is about breaking down the gender binary, and as such, NexUp is committed to listening, learning, and adapting new ways to create spaces that are safer, supportive, and motivating for all trans, two-spirit, gender non-conforming, non-binary, and gender queer individuals of all races, ethnicities, and cultural backgrounds. This means that NexUp welcomes and acknowledges the beauty, knowledge, and lived experience of all gender identities, expressions, and sexualities. As such, it incorporates elements of Connell's true vision and purpose for a plurality of masculinities as applied to men's health program design (Connell & Messerschmidt, 2005).

NexUp builds on the foundational approaches that made DUDES Club so successful and sustainable over the years. This applied evolution of the DUDES Club for younger participants holds great promise for formalizing the power of intergenerational learning and participation.

Policy Implications

We have long considered the DUDES Club to play an advocacy role on behalf of the Indigenous communities that we support. We have been in a position of trusted partner with these communities which has provided us the opportunity to listen, reflect and act in a good way to bring greater attention to the significant challenges that Indigenous communities continue to face in Canada. This process would also likely apply to other marginalised, racialised, and colonised groups in diverse settings around the world. Here are four key policy recommendations that we believe require urgent and sustained attention in partnership with the affected communities:

1. *Advocate for more innovative approaches to wellness that effectively decolonise how the health care system is set up to engage and care for Indigenous and racialised people.* As the health care system is rife with systemic racism that causes many harms, it needs to be replaced with models such as the DUDES Club to invite men to engage with the healthcare system in a positive way, while focusing on the prevention of illness and therapeutic partnerships with healthcare providers. DUDES Club is a noteworthy Canadian example of how governments can realize their commitments to implement the United Nations Declaration Rights of Indigenous Peoples (United Nations, 2007)[3] and TRC Calls to Action in health and beyond.

2. *Support Indigenous-led health partnerships and local Indigenous and community-driven program development.* This can help enhance Indigenous community control in health program design and delivery for Indigenous communities. Relatedly, models of care should be expanded to provide continuous support for people living on and off-reserve and account for the reality that while more than half of Indigenous people live off-reserve and many migrate back and forth (e.g., TRC Call to Action #20, 2015b)

3. *Advocate for more flexible sources of funding that allow for organic, community-responsive programming.* Governments have been improving in this regard, especially since the COVID-19 pandemic. Sustained pressure is required to ensure this novel approach to funding continues to provide greater creativity and responsiveness in program design, delivery and reporting at the community level.

4. *Address men's health with an eye toward community health.* Addressing men's health is one aspect of overall community health and will enrich the future of whole communities when all members are given a place to find safety, trust, and support.

Conclusion

The DUDES Club is a disruptive social innovation primarily because of the disconnection between the mainstream health system and the richness and power of Indigenous wellness practices in Canada. DUDES Club members are recovering practices that have withstood the onslaught of Canada's colonial history. Indigenous ways of knowing and healing are essential in addressing the dire health and social problems wrought by colonialism. When we began sharing the success of the DUDES Club model with various Indigenous communities around British Columbia, the matriarchs and female leaders would often ask "where are our men?", referring specifically to how men had lost their way within themselves and within the community. This question still echoes today, but since the beginning of DUDES Club we have seen, heard, and felt the many ways that DUDES Club members are reclaiming their spirit and their role in community while supporting each other to walk a path of healing. In time, we hope that this question "where are our men?" shifts to a resounding affirmation: "our men are home; healthy and proud sons, uncles, fathers, grandfathers, husbands, partners, and friends." Above all, the connections that DUDES Club members establish with each other, their language, their culture, and the land resonate as the very source of success for this model, and its potential to inspire similarly impactful models in other communities around the world.

Acknowledgments We wish to honour the long-standing support and contributions of our following colleagues, and for their thoughtful edits and comments of the manuscript:

- Dr. David Kuhl, Professor, Faculty of Medicine, University of British Columbia
- Dr. Lyana Patrick, Assistant Professor, Faculty of Health Sciences, Simon Fraser University
- Dr. Victoria Smye, Director and Associate Professor, Arthur Labatt Family School of Nursing, Faculty of Health Sciences, University of Western Ontario

References

Adelson, N. (2005). The embodiment of inequity: Health disparities in aboriginal Canada. *Canadian Journal of Public Health, 96, S45–S61.* https://doi.org/10.1007/BF03403702.

Allan, B., & Smylie, J. (2015). First peoples, second class treatment: The role of racism in the health and Well-being of indigenous peoples in Canada. *Wellesley Institute.* https://www.wellesleyinstitute.com/wp-content/uploads/2015/02/Summary-First-Peoples-Second-Class-Treatment-Final.pdf

Connell, R. W., & Messerschmidt, J. W. (2005). Hegemonic masculinity: Rethinking the concept. *Gender & Society, 19*, 829–859. https://doi.org/10.1177/2F0891243205278639

DUDES Club. (2021). *About.* https://dudesclub.ca/about/

DUDES Club. (n.d.a). *Locations.* https://dudesclub.ca/locations/

DUDES Club. (n.d.b). *Evaluation Report.* https://dudesclub.ca/evaluation-report/#methods

Efimoff, I., Patrick, L., Josewski, V., Gross, P. A., Lambert, S., & Smye, V. (2021). The power of connections: How a novel Canadian men's wellness program is improving the health and well-being of Indigenous and non-Indigenous men. *The International Indigenous Policy Journal, 12(2), 1–22.* https://doi.org/10.18584/iipj.2021.12.2.10896.

Fiola, C., & MacKinnon, S. (2020). Urban and inner-city studies: Decolonizing ourselves and the University of Winnipeg. In S. Cote-Meek & T. Moeke-Pickering (Eds.), *Decolonizing and indigenizing education in Canada (pp. 155–173). Canadian Scholars' Press.*

First Nations Health Authority. (2017). *Overdose data and first nations in BC: Preliminary findings.* https://www.fnha.ca/AboutSite/NewsAndEventsSite/NewsSite/Documents/FNHA_OverdoseDataAndFirstNationsInBC_PreliminaryFindings_FinalWeb_July2017.pdf

Goldenberg, S. L. (2014). Status of men's health in Canada. *Canadian Urological Association Journal, 8(7–8), S142–S144.* https://doi.org/10.5489/cuaj.2308.

Greenwood, M., De Leeuw, S., Lindsay, N. M., & Reading, C. (Eds.). (2015). *Determinants of indigenous peoples' health in Canada: Beyond the social.* Canadian Scholars' Press.

Gross, P. A., Efimoff, I., Patrick, L., Joweski, V., Hau, K., Lambert, S., & Smye, V. (2016). The DUDES Club: A brotherhood for men's health. *Canadian Family Physician, 62*(6), e311–e318.

Henry, B. (2018). *B.C.'s response to the overdose emergency.* https://www.mass.gov/doc/henry-hrc-12-17-2018/download

Krausz, M., & Jang, K. (2015). Lessons from the creation of Canada's poorest postal code. *The Lancet Psychiatry, 2, e5.* https://doi.org/10.1016/S2215-0366(15)00045-0.

King, M., & Gracey, M. (2009). Indigenous health part 2: The underlying causes of the health gap. *The Lancet, 374, 76–85.* https://doi.org/10.1016/S01406736(09)60827-8.

Oliffe, J. L., McCreary, D. R., Black, N., Flannigan, R., & Goldenberg, S. L. (2020a). Canadian men's health literacy: A nationally representative study. *Health Promotion Practice, 21(6), 993–1003.* https://doi.org/10.1177/1524839919837625.

Oliffe, J. L., Rossnagel, E., Bottorff, J. L., Chambers, S. K., Caperchione, C., & Rice, S. M. (2020b). Community-based men's health promotion programs: *Eight lessons learnt and their caveats. Health Promotion International, 35(5), 1230–1240.* https://doi.org/10.1093/heapro/daz101.

Smith, J. A., Christie, B., Bonson, J., Adams, M., Osborne, R., Judd, B., Drummond, M., Aanundsen, D., & Fleay, J. (2019). *Health literacy among young Aboriginal and Torres Strait islander males in the Northern Territory.* Menzies School of Health Research.

Truth and Reconciliation Commission of Canada. (2015a). *Canada's residential schools: The history, part 1 origins to 1939* (Vol. 1). Queen's University Press.

Truth and Reconciliation Commission of Canada. (2015b). *Calls to action.* http://trc.ca/assets/pdf/Calls_to_Action_English2.pdf

Tuck, E., & Yang, K. W. (2012). Decolonization is not a metaphor. *Decolonization: Indigeneity, Education & Society, 1(1), 1–40.* https://jps.library.utoronto.ca/index.php/des/article/view/18630.

United Nations. (2007). *United Nations declaration of the rights of indigenous peoples.* https://www.un.org/en/about-us/universal-declaration-of-human-rights

Chapter 7
Coming to Know Ishkode: Re-Encountering Indigenous Male Wholistic Wellness in Canada

Garrison McCleary

Introduction

Indigenous men in Canada suffer greater health disparities, higher incarceration rates, shorter lifespans, and lower high school graduation rates than their non-Indigenous counterparts (Canuto et al., 2015). As such, Innes and Anderson (2015) rightly ask the question, "who is walking with our brothers?" (Anderson et al., 2015, p. 4). While a growing body of scholarly literature has begun to address issues specific to Indigenous men, research on urban Indigenous masculinities remains in its infancy (Anderson et al., 2015; Bang et al., 2014; Innes & Anderson, 2015; McKegney, 2014). This research is only beginning to scratch the surface of the intersections of race and gender on the expression of healthy and wholistic Indigenous masculinities. Much of this work has focused on rebalancing wholistic wellness (an attention to the balancing of spiritual, emotional, mental, and physical well-being) among Indigenous men through ceremony, teachings, and men's programming (Antone, 2015). However, with a few program exceptions (e.g., I am a Kind Man and The Dudes Club), these places and spaces for Indigenous male healing, community, and intervention continue to remain inaccessible within many urban contexts, especially in therapeutic Land-based formats (e.g., fire keeping, hunting & trapping, fishing, men's outdoor gatherings, and gardening) (Bang et al., 2014; Efimoff et al., 2021; Firestone et al., 2021; Innes & Anderson, 2015; Joe, 2001; Waddell et al., 2021). Through a discussion of wholism and wellness, this chapter will explore Indigenous masculinities, and their interaction with the urban environment. This discussion is situated within the context of the "Building the Fire Project", a community based urban Indigenous male wellness research project in Guelph, Ontario, Canada.

G. McCleary (✉)
Wilfrid Laurier University, Kitchener, Canada
e-mail: gmccleary@wlu.ca

© The Editor(s) (if applicable) and The Author(s), under exclusive license to
Springer Nature Switzerland AG 2023
J. A. Smith et al. (eds.), *Health Promotion with Adolescent Boys and Young Men of Colour*, https://doi.org/10.1007/978-3-031-22174-3_7

Indigenous Masculinities

It is important to begin this chapter by exploring how masculinity is generally conceptualised, as these generalisations often inform the intrapersonal and social relations that contribute to the development of a wholistically well male identity. The Oxford Dictionary vaguely defines masculinity as "the fact of being a man; the qualities that are considered to be typical to men" (Oxford University, 2022). Historically, this definition has used biological sex as the determining factor of the masculine identity. However, much of the contemporary research on gender and critical masculinity studies contradicts this approach by situating gender and masculinity as socially, culturally, and environmentally constructed. Accordingly, this contemporary definition would suggest that expressions of masculinity are unique across contexts and that such qualities of being a "man" are constituted through said contexts (Anderson et al., 2015; Connell & Messerschmidt, 2005). As a result, a dynamic and fluid conceptualization of masculinity has become more prevalent and widely accepted across the literature. This multiplicity of masculinities provides a navigational challenge for all men, including urban Indigenous men, to engage in the healthy development of a wholistic self and male identity within their own contexts.

Urban Indigenous men reside within a colonial reality represented physically by the concrete jungle in which they live. In these urban settler-colonial spaces, the common expressions of masculinity are shrouded in the Euro-Western patriarchy that centres detachment, individualism, and power-over at the centre of the masculine ideal. The social and political processes (e.g., social media, advertising, and business) of white settler society places the white heterosexual male as the perfect specimen of this masculine ideal to which all men must aspire. While this ideal boasts of fulfilment and satisfaction, it is unattainable within the social practice reality of men – especially men of colour (Davis, 1981; hooks, 2004). While the promises of life fulfilment and satisfaction associated with this masculine ideal often go unfulfilled, men, nevertheless continue to benefit from the patriarchal system irrespective of class, race, sexual orientation, and location. However, intersectional identities complicate this simplistic understanding of patriarchy and provide an intra-gender understanding of both privilege and disadvantage within this gender group (Carbado et al., 2013; Collins, 1998; Crenshaw, 1989; Haywood et al., 2018; Tayler et al., 2010).

Accordingly, Indigenous men are caught at the intersections of male privilege and racial exclusion (Connell & Messerschmidt, 2005; Malton, 2019). While in many ways still benefiting from the Euro-Western patriarchal system, Indigenous men struggle to find space to articulate an understanding of their own masculine ideal that challenges Euro-Western patriarchal customs and recentres cultural practices and understandings of masculinity (Innes & Anderson, 2015; Malton, 2019; Norman et al., 2019). In navigating this intersectional place, Indigenous men are looking to their culture, kinship structures, and traditional Land-based practices for direction in redefining an Indigenous masculine ideal (Anderson et al., 2015; Thunderbird Partnership Foundation, 2020). Innes and Anderson (2015) highlight the entrenched responsibilities and relationships that describe an Indigenous mascu-linity. These responsibilities and relationships intertwined between the Land, family and community provide a backdrop for how Indigenous men are navigating the intersections of gender and race (Innes & Anderson, 2015). While many of their research participants struggled and often refused to define Indigenous masculinity, there remained a deep understanding of how entrenched colonial practices inform the assertion of white masculinity over Indigenous men. This assertion, and the often violent acceptance of white masculinity by Indigenous men, consequently damages the responsibilities and relationships many Indigenous men seek to reclaim (Innes & Anderson, 2015; McKegney, 2014). Traversing these spaces highlights the many barriers Indigenous men face in redefining what it is to be a wholistically well man.

Wholistic Wellness

The two interconnected concepts of wholism and wellness within an Indigenous context are central to understanding how a wholistically well Indigenous male iden-tity is developed and embodied. A brief discussion on wholism and the Anishinaabe Medicine Wheel will be presented, followed by a definition of well-ness within an Indigenous framework. It must be noted that while the direc-tional concepts of wholism (Anishinaabe Medicine Wheel) and wellness have been separated for the descriptive benefit of the reader, these concepts are inseparable and reliant upon one another (Hill, 2014, 2020; Kennedy-Kish et al., 2017; Absolon, 2010; Nabigon, 2006.

Wholism

Many definitions of wholism are grounded in traditional teachings from Indigenous nations across Turtle Island (North America). Hill (2020) provides one general defi-nition: "wholism refers to the inherent interconnection with the earth and all the spirits of the Creation" (p. 8). While brief, this definition reminds us that across contexts and populations, the process of working towards wholism involves the full-ness of Creation including that which is beyond human. This is an important distinc-tion as it provides an understanding of how urban Indigenous male wholism does not occur within a vacuum; rather it exists within larger communal (human and non-human) contexts. Entrenched in this understanding is the deep and interrelated connection human beings have with Creation. This understanding is especially important when discussing the wholistic needs of urban Indigenous populations who have often been dislocated from these natural places where these connections have been traditionally and historically nurtured (Bang et al., 2014; Hatala et al., 2020; Innes & Anderson, 2015; Waddell et al., 2021).Wholism can also refer to the balance and harmony of all four aspects of self as outlined through the cardinal directions of the Anishinaabe Medicine Wheel. (Absolon, 2010; Hill, 2014, 2016, 2020; Kennedy-Kish et al., 2017; Nabigon, 2006; Nabigon & Mawhiney, 1996).

Anishinaabe Medicine Wheel

The Anishinaabe Medicine Wheel is a contemporary and central circular symbol of wholism (Absolon, 2010; Graveline, 1998; Hill, 2014, 2016, 2020; Hill & Cooke, 2014; Kennedy-Kish et al., 2017; Nabigon, 2006; Nabigon & Mawhiney, 1996; Norman et al., 2019). It includes, but is not limited to, "the interrelationship between different aspects of creation, and cycle of life, as well as everything else that comprises the worldviews of Indigenous peoples" (Hill, 2020, p. 8). It is most often; however, not exclusively, divided into the cardinal directions or four quadrants starting in the East (Spiritual) moving to the South (Emotional), to the West (Mental), and then the North (Physical) (Absolon, 2010; Hill, 2014; Kennedy-Kish et al., 2017). Frequently, the Medicine Wheel is used as a tool to engage a lifelong process of seeking wholistic balance. This chapter will focus on the Anishinaabe Medicine Wheel as described by Hill (2008, 2016, 2020), Hill & Cooke (2014). It should be noted that there remains many iterations and directional teachings associated with the Medicine Wheel which are not included within the following discussion.

Eastern Direction

The Eastern direction of the Anishinaabe Medicine Wheel is representative of the spiritual self, beginnings, teachings, and rebirth (Absolon, 2010; Hill, 2014, 2016, 2020; Kennedy-Kish et al, 2017). In this direction, one engages with a "personal, deep, inner connection with the Creator and all of Creation" (Hill, 2020, p. 27). This spirit connection should be nurtured and protected as individuals walk on their physical journey (Absolon, 2010; Hill, 2020; Kennedy-Kish et al., 2017; Nabigon, 2006; Nabigon & Mawhiney, 1996). Hill (2020) notes that it is in this direction that individuals must learn how to honour their spirit. Ceremonies, celebrations (such as harvest gatherings), and other rituals have been used by Indigenous peoples to nurture these spiritual relationships. Urban manicured parks and naturalized spaces provide a unique challenge to urban Indigenous people in maintaining their connection with Creation. Particularly, urban Indigenous men cannot engage traditional hunting and fishing practices within city limits, interrupting a spiritual connection with the animals, fish, and ceremonies that often generate meaning, self-awareness, and community inclusion (Bang et al., 2014; Hatala et al., 2020; Waddell et al., 2021). However, urban practices such as walking, hiking, bird watching, container gardening, and urban community ceremonies and celebrations (e.g., Sacred Fires), can help urban Indigenous men continue to make these important spiritual connections to Creation, each other, and themselves.

Southern Direction

The Southern direction of the Anishinaabe Medicine Wheel is representative of the emotional self and relationships (Absolon, 2010; Hill, 2014, 2016, 2020; Kennedy-Kish et al., 2017; Nabigon, 2006). Our emotions are what animate our relationship to Creation (human and non-human), and as such, must be nurtured, expressed, and released regularly (Hill, 2020; Kennedy-Kish et al., 2017; Nabigon & Mawhiney, 1996; Thunderbird Partnership Foundation, 2020). In many ways, coopted by the Western patriarchy, Indigenous men have been taught and told to detach from their emotions. This detachment fulfills the "Stoic Indian" stereotype that the Western world continues to assert (Mihseuah, 1996). However, there is an increasing amount of literature examining shifts in positive emotional expression within homosocial relationships that challenge these notions (Haywood et al., 2018). This exemplifies a potential shift in the toxic masculine narrative that is prevalent within the current homogenous society. For example, emerging research on the roles of Indigenous fathers in re-learning of positive emotional expression and nurturance are signifying a shift in how Indigenous men are reclaiming emotions as a space for positive relational building (Ball, 2010). This shift in understanding and practice is extremely important for urban Indigenous men, especially young men, attempting to establish a balanced life.

Western Direction

The Western direction of the Anishinaabe Medicine Wheel is representative of the mental self and knowledge (Absolon, 2010; Hill & Cooke, 2014; Kennedy-Kish, et al., 2017). This encompasses our ability to reflect and articulate our ideas and thoughts to uncover meaning within our personal lives, our work, and our relationships. (Hill, 2020; Kennedy-Kish et al., 2017). Through this constant process of reflecting and articulating of our experiences, we come to acquire embodied wisdom (Hill, 2020). As human-beings we are able to think and reflect on our responsibilities to ourselves and all our relations which enables us to understand the transformation or healing we need to seek balance and harmony within our lives and relationships (Hill, 2014, 2016 2020; Nabigon & Mawhiney, 1996). For urban Indigenous men, awareness of over-stimulation in the urban space through media, noise, or advertising is important, as these stimulants can disrupt reflective processes and the ability to articulate important ideas and thoughts about their life path

(Hill, 2020). There remains many barriers for urban Indigenous men to connect with Elders, Knowledge Keepers, and mentors in urban spaces. These individuals provide important support in developing wholistic self through fasting, vision quests, reflective processes, critical self-awareness, and other ceremonies and rituals.

Northern Direction

The Northern direction of the Anishinaabe Medicine Wheel is representative of the physical self, doing, and movement (Absolon, 2010; Hill & Cooke, 2014; Kennedy-Kish et al, 2017). Many Indigenous peoples see the body as the physical vessel for Spirit to be present in this physical world (Benton-Banai, 1988; Hill, 2014, 2016, 2020; Kennedy-Kish et al., 2017; Nabigon, 2006; Nabigon & Mawhiney, 1996). Our bodies allow us to interpret and understand when we feel illness caused by an imbalance in one or more of the other three aspects of self: spiritual, emotional, and mental as outlined within the Medicine Wheel. Hill (2020) states that the "physical self, being the indicator of imbalance and disharmony, requires special attention and constant monitoring" (p. 33). Hill further indicates that our bodies' health is contingent on four things: hydration, breathing, diet, and exercise (Hill, 2016, 2020). To attend to the physical aspects of self, a cultivated awareness of embodied reactions and responses to external and internal stimulants (e.g., stomach aches and back pain) is needed (Hill, 2020). For many urban Indigenous men struggling to live a traditional lifestyle, physical wellness provides a space for men to engage in socially accepted health behaviours such as going to the gym, healthy eating, and drinking water. However, it should be noted that engagement with healthy behaviours, such as those indicated above, does not equate to wholistic balance – rather, the physical self can act as an intentional entry point to deeper engagement with the other aspects of self.

Again, it is important to note that while each of these aspects of self are described in subsections of this chapter, each quadrant is of equal value and must be regularly nurtured when seeking wholistic balance. In working towards wholistic balance, Indigenous men must recognize that there is no end point in which they reach full balance; rather it is the process and journey towards balance and wellness that is of importance. In the constant striving for balance, Indigenous men incrementally become more wholistically well for themselves, their families, and their communities.

Wellness

While there are many definitions of wellness, I have chosen to include the definition outlined by the Thunderbird Partnership Foundation and Elder Onaubinisay (Jim Dumont). It provides a culturally congruent definition and framework applicable to practice with many Indigenous people. Consistent with the previous section on wholism, wellness is defined by the Thunderbird Partnership Foundation (2020) as:

> …a whole and healthy person expressed through a sense of balance of spirit, emotion, mind and body. Central to wellness is belief in one's connection to language, Land, beings of creation, and ancestry, supported by a caring family and environment. The spirit causes us to live, gives us vitality, mobility, purpose and the desire to achieve the highest quality of living in the world (p. 4).

Engaging Indigenous wellness can be extremely challenging for urban Indigenous men as they are often severed from the very connections that are central to their wellness. Facilitated rebuilding of these relational pathways for urban Indigenous men are needed to address the challenges of urban Indigenous social determinants of health. The "Building the Fire Project" is one such program that was envisioned to do just that.

Building the Fire Project

The "Building the Fire Project" was a community-based research project conducted in Guelph, Ontario, Canada between the spring of 2018 to the summer of 2019. The project sought to provide an inter-generational space for urban Indigenous men and male identified individuals, to gather, share, and build community. The project was headed by Dr. Kim Anderson (Cree/Metis), Canada Research Chair in Indigenous Relationships and Associate Professor in the Department of Family Relations and Applied Nutrition in the College of Social and Applied Human Sciences at the University of Guelph, and Dr. Robert Innes (Plains Cree), Associate Professor in the Department of Native Studies at the University of Saskatchewan. Rob Baldwin, Dr. Cara Wehkamp, and multiple young Indigenous male Oshkaabewis' (helpers), including the author, served as members of the larger research team. While Dr. Anderson was nominated primary investigator on the project, the fire gathering activities were open to men or male identifying individuals only.

This project was funded through the Canadian Institute for Health Research (CIHR) and grounded in Indigenous concepts of wholistic wellness, keeping with the Institute of Aboriginal People's Health mandate. The project was originally intended to be intergenerational, focusing specifically on having young urban Indigenous men from the three local universities engage with older urban Indigenous men in a sacred Land-based space, offering bi-weekly fire circles, traditional men's teachings, and one-on-one support for health and wellness along the way. However, due to limited attendance by the younger demographic, participation was opened to all urban Indigenous men in the community irrespective of age. The circles were facilitated by Rob Baldwin, an "Uncle" of the Aboriginal Resource Centre at the University of Guelph, and an experienced counsellor with a longstanding practice and interest in men's mental health. It is important to note that circle process includes the facilitator as an active and equal participant within the circle.

This research was informed by Indigenous health concepts grounded in the interconnection and well-being of "all our relations". This includes intergenerational human relations and relations to the Land and to the past and future generations in the form of ancestral/spirit relations. The goal of the project was to foster Indigenous men's wellness according to this wholistic approach. In this way, healthy aging for Indigenous peoples was about moving beyond serving an aging demographic in isolation to improving health and relations for and between different generations of Indigenous men and nurturing how these generational connections with the natural world and spirit come into being.

A men's fire circle was chosen for this project in light of evidence that previous programs connecting Indigenous men and fire have had positive outcomes (Antone, 2015), and that Land-based approaches to research and learning have proven to be very effective in conveying Indigenous perspectives (Bang et al., 2014; Hatala et al., 2020; Thunderbird Partnership Foundation, 2020; Waddell et al., 2021; Wildcat et al., 2014). For many Indigenous cultures, fire opens the doorway to spirit so that spirit can be present in the healing relationship. Fire can be used as a teaching tool about life balance and support healthy mastery of important life skills such as relational and social communication and emotional awareness. The circle of men situated around the fire collectively helped build confidence, self-esteem, and a sense of belonging between each other. The training of Ohskabewis in leadership roles, circle leading, and fire keeping were seen as key to knowledge translation post research project.

Ultimately, this research intended to contribute knowledge about Land-based spaces that can support urban Indigenous men's health and wholistic wellness across the life span. The project was set to conclude with a small gathering of facilitators, knowledge carriers, and end users who are creating spaces for intergenerational Indigenous men's health and wellness in other post-secondary institutions across Canada. At the writing of this chapter, the event has yet to take place due to the public health measures enacted due to the COVID-19 pandemic.

Methodology

Participation in the project was open to Indigenous men and male identifying individuals who lived within local communities surrounding the Sacred Fire sites (Guelph-Wellington and Kitchener-Waterloo- Cambridge regions). The participant group was comprised of 10 men; however, most gatherings averaged 5–6 men. One of the participants was a trans man, while the rest of the participants were cisgendered Indigenous men. Two non-Indigenous participants were also permitted to participate in the project as they had close connections both personally and professionally to the local Indigenous community. The participants ages ranged from early 20s to late 70s. The project participants convened bi-weekly at one of two sites: one located in a more rural setting on the edge of town, and the second located along the Speed River which runs through the heart of the City of Guelph's downtown core.

Regional Elders and Knowledge Carriers were welcomed monthly to share their knowledge with the men around the Sacred Fire. Most of the circles were well attended; however, sometimes only a few men participated due to inclement weather, work commitments, or personal/family matters.

The research team recorded seven semi-structured interviews: three with the project facilitator and four with the project's Knowledge Carriers, before and after their participation in the circles. One participant submitted notes in response to the research questions. These interviews focused on the participants' general reflections to capture how they experienced wellness during the project and what else they thought might support wellness for Indigenous men in future projects or gatherings. The interviews and notes were transcribed and then a thematic analysis was conducted by the research team using inductive coding in N-Vivo (Braun & Clarke, 2006).

Reflection on Men's Voices

The following subsections provide reflections on the participants' interviews conducted for the project, including three themes that emerged from the data analysis. While this chapter discusses only three emergent themes from the research, they nevertheless hold value in understanding how this kind of project may impact the development of future programming for urban Indigenous male wholistic wellness.

Fire at the Centre

All the participants in the project highlighted the importance of having a physical fire during these sharing circles and teachings. Many of the participants spoke about the centrality of the fire to the project and the gifts that the fire passed to them. The presence of the fire brought an extra level of intentionality to the work. This was exemplified by one participant's comment about the fire when he was asked about how the program engaged men in wellness: "Well, I should say…being around the fire…being facilitated around the fire as well, right? In the sense that we're not just hanging out around the fire." This participant notes how Rob and the Ohskabewis' created the space for the intentionality and sacredness of the work (i.e., building the fire, lighting the fire, and the sharing circles or teachings with other men). Many participants acknowledged that the fire was important, but it was not until they could feel the presence of the fire working within them and within the other participants in the group that they really began to understand the nature of its role in facilitating the opening of a doorway to healing.

There is large body of literature in critical masculinity studies that examines how homosocial relationships between men often continue to support and maintain homogenous masculinity and patriarchy. However, like the arguments presented by

Haywood et al. (2018), the homosocial behaviour illustrated between men within the "Building the Fire Project" indicate a dissention from homogenous masculinity (p. 59). These homosocial relationships, which emerged through collaboration and intimate sharing between men, actively challenge the dominant homogenous masculinity. By doing so they instead begin to redefine and promote an Indigenous masculinity through the transformation of rigid gender binaries, male intimacy, and power relations.

This transformative process can be seen in how many men within the project engaged in spiritual and emotional openness about their own wholistic journey. One participant noted the connections and inspiration he felt about his own path when participating at the fires:

> I feel like I have a really bright fire that guides me in my heart, and being around that fire is tremendous inspiration, and when I say my prayers in the morning to the sun right out my window, I think about that fire. The sun's fire being in the fire circle and that its all connecting me to keep enlivening and keep encouraging me to put one foot in front of the other. I don't have a big plan. It's like what are my ancestors revealing to me?

While it is evident that this participant had a clear idea of what he was receiving from these gatherings, he exemplifies how the Sacred Fire is encountered with an unknowingness of the healing or gifts being sought. Through the intimate relationship with the Sacred Fire and with the other men around the circle, one comes closer to knowing the vision or direction of their wholistic wellness journey. These connections and relationships also tease out the responsibilities that define their Indigenous masculinity.

Connection

The gatherings hosted through the project allowed men to come to know one another in an intergenerational setting on the Land. Many of the older men, Elders, and Knowledge Keepers that participated in the project had been on their wellness and healing journeys for a long time. They provided reflections and wisdom to the younger participants on navigating relationships, self-worth, employment, and emotions such as sadness, anger, and grief. One participant noted the uniqueness of this process:

> I have other healthy male relationships, but we don't often sit around the fire and talk, you know. It's really rare. On a fishing trip or canoe trip you kind of do that but it's never intentional. So, having it as intentional is really, really good. And I think that you kind of throw off your day, or even kind of, typically the busyness of your day, and then [inaudible] or of your week, or of your month or whatever. And you have time to kind of just listen.

It is important to acknowledge how men came together during these sharing circles in a vulnerable and open way. The uniqueness and rarity of the tender moments between men that were experienced during these circles are a testament to how the Land and Sacred Fire can facilitate powerful connections and bonds. Being surrounded by healthy and loving men can help one to become less judgmental of oneself, and to embrace the unfolding process of coming into one's wellness journey in a kind and loving way.

Engagement

Engagement of Indigenous men in wellness programming can be challenging as the dominant culture continues to value the toxic masculine ideals espoused by Western patriarchy. Many of the men struggled to be open and vulnerable when they first attended the project circles, first with others, and then with themselves. However, many participants noted that the challenges of engaging men should not be a justification for not offering programming; instead it affirms that programming is needed. One participant stated, "if you build it, they will come," highlighting both the need for and scarcity of existing Indigenous men's programming in the region. This notion was further supported by another participant who spoke about the slow development of a "central core" of men who were dedicated and intentional in their participation in the Sacred Fire circles:

> Yeah, there seems to be a central core that is developing. And it has taken a while for that to happen, and that's okay, we've kind of anticipated that. I think part of the process is being willing to stick around. Like you said, to show up. And putting the energy out there and inviting them to come even though it's still happening.

Men who became the "central core" of the circles provided the "Building the Fire Project" with a platform for the future development or mobilization of similar programming for other urban Indigenous men in the future.

The small group of men that engaged with this project were intentional and committed to doing healing work for themselves, their families, and their communities. While the research component of this project has concluded, a group of men continues to gather and share with one another around the Sacred Fire. This is testament to the transformative nature of these programs on the development of healthy and wholistic pathways for urban Indigenous men.

Conclusion

Many urban Indigenous men struggle to navigate their intersectional location and find it difficult to enact an Indigenous masculinity when the dominant masculine ideal is in direct opposition. The dislocation from Land and ceremonies that has come with the urbanization of Indigenous peoples has magnified health disparities. Institutional and infrastructural barriers such as city bylaws, urban planning, fire regulations, and labour-intensive bureaucratic approval processes limit the establishment of Sacred Fire spaces for men's wellness and healing in the urban setting.

Despite these barriers, we can begin to unpack and rebuild Indigenous masculinities and their interactions within the urban environment through applying the concepts of wholism and wellness, and a deeper understanding of how such concepts interact within homosocial relationships. The "Men's Building the Fire Project" helped to illuminate these processes in action, and now exists as a potential program blueprint for the development of future urban Indigenous male wellness programming.

References

Absolon, K. (2010). Indigenous wholistic theory: A knowledge set for practice. *First Peoples Child and Family Review, 14*(1), 74–87.

Anderson, K., Swift, J., & Innes, R. (2015). "To arrive speaking": Voices from the Bidwewidam indigenous masculinities project. In R. Innes & K. Anderson (Eds.), *Indigenous men and masculinities: Legacies, identities, regeneration* (pp. 283–307). University of Manitoba Press.

Antone, B. (2015). Reconstructing indigenous masculine thought. In R. Innes & K. Anderson (Eds.), *Indigenous Men and Masculinities: Legacies, Identities, Regeneration* (pp. 21–37). University of Manitoba Press.

Ball, J. (2010). Indigenous fathers' involvement in reconstituting "circles of care". *American Journal of Community Psychology, 45*(1), 124–138. https://doi.org/10.1007/s10464-009-9293-1

Bang, M., Curley, L., Kessel, A., Marin, A., & Iii, S. S. (2014). Muskrat theories, tobacco in the streets, and living Chicago as indigenous land. *Environmental Education Research*, 1–19. https://doi.org/10.1080/13504622.2013.865113

Benton-Banai, E. (1988). *The Mishomis book: The voice of the Ojibway.* University of Minnesota Press.

Braun, V., & Clarke, V. (2006). Using thematic analysis in psychology. *Qualitative Research in Psychology, 3*(2), 77–101. https://doi.org/10.1191/1478088706qp063oa

Canuto, K., Brown, A., Harfield, S., & Wittert, G. (2015). Strategies that target the utilization of primary health care services by indigenous men in Australia, New Zealand, Canada and America: A comprehensive systematic review protocol. *JBI Database of Systematic Reviews and Implementation Reports, 13*(9), 95–111. https://doi.org/10.11124/jbisrir-2015-2319

Carbado, D. W., Crenshaw, K. W., Mays, V. M., & Tomlinson, B. (2013). Intersectionality: Mapping the movements of a theory. *Du Bois Review, 10*(2), 303–312. https://doi.org/10.1017/S1742058X13000349

Collins, P. H. (1998). It's all in the family: Intersections of gender, race and nation. *Hypatia1, 13*(3), 62–82.

Connell, R. W., & Messerschmidt, J. W. (2005). Hegemonic masculinity rethinking the concept. *Gender and Society, 19*(6), 829–859. https://doi.org/10.1177/0891243205278639

Crenshaw, K. W. (1989). Demarginalizing the intersection of race and sex: A black feminist critique of anti-discrimination doctrine, feminist theory and antiracist politics. *University of Chicago Legal Forum, 1989*(1), 139–167.

Davis, A. (1981). *Women, race, and class.* Vintage Books.

Efimoff, I., Patrick, L., Josewski, V., Gross, P., Lambert, S., & Smye, V. (2021). Power of connections: How a novel Canadian men's wellness program is improving the health and Well-being of indigenous and non-indigenous men. *International Indigenous Policy Journal, 12*(2), 1–22. https://doi.org/10.18584/iipj.2021.12.2.10896

Firestone, M., Syrette, J., Brant, T., Laing, M., & Teekens, S. (2021). Findings from a process evaluation of an indigenous holistic housing support and mental health case management program in downtown Toronto. *International Journal of Indigenous Health, 16*(2), 139–151. https://doi.org/10.32799/ijih.v16i2.33173

Graveline, F. J. (1998). *Circle works: Transforming Eurocentric consciousness*. Fernwood Publishing.

Hatala, A., Njese, C., Morton, D., Pearl, T., & Bird-Naytohow, K. (2020). Land and nature as sources of health and resilience among indigenous youth in an urban Canadian context: A photovoice exploration. *BMC Public Health, 20*(538), 1–14.

Haywood, C., Johanssen, T., Hammarén, N., Hertz, M., & Ottemo, A. (2018). Homosociality: Misogyny, fraternity and new intimacies. In *The conundrum of masculinity: Hegemony, homosociality, homophobia, and hetereonormativity* (pp. 56–76). Routledge.

Hill, L. (2008). Understanding Indigenous Canadian traditional health and healing. In ProQuest Dissertations and Theses.

Hill, G. (2014). *A holistic aboriginal framework for individual healing* (pp. 59–69). Cure of the soul.

Hill, G. & Cooke, M. (2014). How do you build a community? Developing community capacity and social capital in an urban aboriginal setting. *Pimatisiwin, 11*(3), 421–432.

Hill, G. (2016). In the trenches: Traditional healers' understanding of health and healing. *Indigenous Social Work Journal., 10*(1), 19–32.

Hill, G. (2020). *Indigenous healing: Voices of elders and healers*. Charlton Publishing.

hooks, B. (2004). *The will to change: Men, masculinity, and love*. Washington Square Press.

Innes, R., & Anderson, K. (2015). *Indigenous men and masculinities: Legacies, identities, regeneration*. University of Manitoba Press.

Joe, J. (2001). Out of harmony: Health problems and young native American men. *Journal of American College Health, 49*(1), 237–242.

Kennedy-Kish, B., Sinclair, R., Carniol, B., & Baines, D. (2017). *Case critical: Social services and social justice in Canada* (7th ed.). Between The Lines.

Malton, J. (2019). *Black masculinity under racial capitalism*. Boston Review.

McKegney, S. (Ed.). (2014). *Masculindians: Conversations about indigenous manhood*. Michigan State University Press.

Mihseuah, D. (1996). *American Indians: Stereotypes & reality*. Clarity Press.

Nabigon, H. (2006). *The hollow tree: Fighting addiction with traditional native healing*. Queen's University Press.

Nabigon, H., & Mawhiney, A. M. (1996). Aboriginal theory: A Cree medicine wheel guide for healing nations. In F. J. Turner (Ed.), *Social work treatment: Interlocking theoretical approaches* (pp. 18–38). The Free Press.

Norman, M. E., Hart, M. A., Petherick, L., McRae, H., Mason, G., Cote, A., Cote, S., & Sinclair, C. (2019). Bringing the 'other half' back: A place-specific intergenerational exploration of indigenous physical cultural masculinities in Fisher River Cree nation. *Qualitative Research in Sport, Exercise and Health, 11*(5), 671–686. https://doi.org/10.1080/2159676X.2018.1510431

Oxford University. (2022). Oxford learners dictionary. https://www.oxfordlearnersdictionaries.com/definition/english/masculinity

Tayler, Y., Hines, S., & Casey, M. (2010). *Theorizing intersectionality and sexuality*. Palgrave Macmillan.

Thunderbird Partnership Foundation. (2020). Indigenous wellness framework reference guide. https://www.thunderbirdpf.org/IWF

Waddell, C. M., de Jager, M. D., Gobeil, J., Tacan, F., Herron, R. V., Allan, J. A., & Roger, K. (2021). Healing journeys: Indigenous men's reflections on resources and barriers to mental wellness. *Social Science and Medicine, 270*(January), 113696. https://doi.org/10.1016/j.socscimed.2021.113696

Wildcat, M., McDonald, M., Irlbacher-Fox, S., & Coulthard, G. (2014). Learning from the land: Indigenous land-based pedagogy and decolonization. *Decolonization: Indigeneity, Education & Society, 3*(3), I–XV.

Chapter 8
Exploring the Social and Cultural Determinants of Indigenous Males' Participation and Success in Higher Education in Australia

Samuel Moore, James A. Smith, Himanshu Gupta, Garth Stahl, Bep Uink, Braden Hill, Jesse J. Fleay, Daile L. Rung, Andrew Harvey, and Peter Radoll

Introduction: Background

Educational systems place multiple constraints on Indigenous people participating and achieving in higher education (Behrendt et al., 2012; Shankar et al., 2013; Frawley Smith & Larkin, 2015; Smith et al., 2017; Wood et al., 2019). University enrolments and course completions for Indigenous Australians have improved in recent years. For example, there was a 90% increase (from 11,024 to 21,033) and more than a doubling (108% increase from 1424 to 2964) in the number

S. Moore · J. A. Smith (✉) · H. Gupta
Freemasons Centre for Male Health and Wellbeing – Northern Territory, Menzies School of Health Research, Charles Darwin University, Darwin, NT, Australia

Rural and Remote Health, College of Medicine and Public Health, Flinders University, Darwin, NT, Australia
e-mail: sam.moore@menzies.edu.au; james.smith@flinders.edu.au

G. Stahl
School of Education, University of Queensland, Brisbane, QLD, Australia
e-mail: g.stahl@uq.edu.au

B. Uink
Kulbardi Aboriginal Centre, Murdoch University, Murdoch, WA, Australia
e-mail: buink@murdoch.edu.au

B. Hill
Centre of Kurongkurl Katitjin, Edith Cowan University, Mt Lawley, WA, Australia
e-mail: b.hill@ecu.edu.au

J. J. Fleay
School of Education, Curtin University, Bentley, WA, Australia
e-mail: j.fleay@curtin.edu.au

© Menzies School of Health Research, the rights holder, and The Editor(s) (if applicable) and The Author(s), under exclusive license to Springer Nature Switzerland AG 2023
J. A. Smith et al. (eds.), *Health Promotion with Adolescent Boys and Young Men of Colour*, https://doi.org/10.1007/978-3-031-22174-3_8

of Indigenous university enrolments and completions between 2010 and 2019, respectively (Department of Education, Skills and Employment, 2020). However, despite this progress, Indigenous Australians continue to be underrepresented in universities making up only 2% of the higher education population in 2019, while representing 3.3% of Australia's total population.

Previous research findings highlight self-efficacy as a powerful driver of success in higher education among Indigenous Australians more generally (Frawley et al., 2017b). Findings show a need for universities to be welcoming and culturally safe spaces, invest in growing the Indigenous academic workforce, embed Indigenous focused curricula within courses, and increase Indigenous support staff based on campus (Buckskin & Tranthim-Fryer, 2018; Pechenkina et al., 2011; Robertson et al., 2021; Smith & Robertson, 2020). Indigenous students, particularly those from remote places, often have family and cultural needs that can create a conflict of responsibilities when they need to travel to major cities for university, often leaving family behind (Rochecouste et al., 2017; Smith et al., 2018).

When we adopt a gender lens, we know that Indigenous males are far less likely to engage in university than Indigenous females (1:3 ratio) (Shalley et al., 2019; Smith et al., 2017; Tomaszewski et al., 2018). This mirrors patterns noted among young Black males in the US (see Chap. 4). Given the cumulative impacts of gender, race and remoteness, Indigenous males enrolment, participation, and completion rates in higher education are a major concern; with emerging evidence suggesting that educational interventions aimed at reducing disengagement and attrition from school and higher education can yield wide-ranging benefits for young Indigenous males across their lifecourse (Australian Institute of Health and Welfare, 2012; Australian Indigenous HealthInfoNet, 2018; Smith, 2018). Yet, there is currently little evidence about what the key characteristics of such interventions might entail. This requires a deeper understanding of the higher education aspirations of young Indigenous males, and the factors promoting higher education participation and achievement of young adult Indigenous males. In tandem, it is important to understand the broader social and economic benefits that extend far beyond the higher education sector (Gupta et al., 2021). For example, the Australian Government *National Men's Health Strategy 2020–2030* identifies that education across the life course is a critical social determinant of health (Department of Health, 2019). In

D. L. Rung
Freemasons Centre for Male Health and Wellbeing – Northern Territory, Menzies School of Health Research, Charles Darwin University, Darwin, NT, Australia
e-mail: daile.rung@cdu.edu.au

A. Harvey
School of Education, Griffith University, Logan, QLD, Australia
e-mail: Andrew.harvey@griffith.edu.au

P. Radoll
People and Organisation, Victoria University, Melbourne, VIC, Australia
e-mail: peter.radoll@vu.edu.au

addition, the cultural determinants of health such as connection to Country,[1] and culture and knowledge systems, are protective factors that positively influence the social determinants of health, including education (Lowitja Institute, 2014; Smith et al., 2018). To support Indigenous students' success at university, these social and cultural connections must be maintained. This will help to reduce health and social inequities experienced by young Indigenous males (Smith et al., 2019, 2020).

Our recent research project funded by the National Centre for Student Equity in Higher Education — entitled *Higher Education Aspirations, Participation, and Achievement of Australian Indigenous males* — aimed to fill this evidence gap (Smith et al., 2022). This chapter presents empirical evidence from this study.

Methods

This chapter draws on qualitative, in-depth semi-structured interviews with 18 Indigenous male higher education students and alumni (aged 18–30) throughout 2020. The participants were from five Australian state and territories (Northern Territory, Western Australia, Victoria, Australian Capital Territory and Queensland) to gain insights into participants' aspirations for, and engagement and participation in, higher education. This chapter includes perspectives from students and alumni based in Alice Springs (Arrernte), Perth (Noongar), Melbourne (Wurundjeri), Bendigo (Dja Dja Wurrung and Taurngurung), Canberra (Ngunnawal) and Brisbane (Turrbal and Jagera). Ethics approval was granted by the Northern Territory Department of Health and Menzies School of Health Research Human Research Ethics Committee (HREC) (2019–3531). Reciprocal ethics approvals were subsequently obtained from the respective HRECs of other participating universities in the remaining four jurisdictions before data collection commenced.

The research team deployed decolonising methodologies and collaborated with multiple Aboriginal and Torres Strait Islander scholars and educators (working in higher education settings) across Australia. Although this project was non-Indigenous led, Indigenous perspectives and attempts to adopt Indigenous Data Sovereignty[2] principles were at the forefront of this research, where research benefits and methods were determined by Indigenous stakeholders (Lovett et al., 2019; Walter & Suina, 2019). This chapter provides an overview of the study's key findings and discusses their implications for policy and practice. The results are clustered into three broad categories: motivations and aspirations to study; higher education engagement and retention barriers; and factors influencing study engagement and success.

---

[1] 'Country' in this context refers to the traditional lands of Indigenous peoples in Australia.

[2] We acknowledge that Indigenous Data Sovereignty is contested terrain and that gaps currently exist between theory and practice. We also acknowledge that this project reflects a collaborative between Indigenous and non-Indigenous researchers, which limits the extent to which IDS can be achieved. Where possible, we used the key principles outlined in the Maiam nayri Wingara Indigenous Data Sovereignty Collective communique to guide our research process (https://www.maiamnayriwingara.org/key-principles)

Results

Motivations and Aspirations to Study

Higher Education Aspirations

The journey to higher education for Indigenous males is shaped by early educational experiences in primary and high school settings. However, the reported lack of engagement in education among Indigenous males needs to be understood in the context of racism and multiple forms of discrimination (both implicit and explicit) experienced in these settings, which can create dispassionate and negative attitudes towards learning.

> There's so many things that are going on prior to walking into university. Like, first of all, to improve it, you need to improve high school standards. You need to improve primary school even. You need to enforce like ... not enforce, but wanting to be lifelong learners. Don't feel like they're being discriminated within the primary and secondary setting before you even get to university. That's how you're going to get them in the door *(Brisbane, studying for undergraduate degree).*

Few of the participants we talked to planned to attend university; instead they planned to pursue work opportunities or Vocational Educational and Training (VET) opportunities, often returning to university later in life.

> I was going to do something like landscape design or something like that at TAFE [Technical and Further Education]. Hopefully do some bricklaying and try and — I was always a little bit more academic and I was going to use that type of side, so I was going to look at architecture and stuff like that. And I was sort of still in that building field. And then after a while I just decided that it was all too hard for me. It was flack knack, I was getting sunburnt, it was exhausting. And, yeah it was, I just decided, look, I don't really think this is going to be me. *(Bendigo, studying for undergraduate degree).*
>
> I've got younger brothers — the indigenous culture or subculture here don't have the aspirations to attend university... There's no leader in there saying that, "You don't have to just go be a tradesman or working in customer service. You can do these other intellectually inclined roles, if you want to, and there is a pathway and there is a road to get there... For example, I know around here, in my brothers' generation, there is probably going to be one Indigenous kid that's going to probably take the leap into university. *(Canberra, studying for undergraduate degree).*

Once engaged in undergraduate degrees, the concept of lifelong learning often flourished, with some students aspiring to achieve postgraduate qualifications to develop more specialised skills:

> I also do have ideas of where I might come back to uni, or if I want to stay on and do uni, like do my masters in teaching, potentially, is an idea I've got. Then another one is doing paramedicine, and like wilderness medicine and that sort of stuff, is another avenue that I'm also very interested in and considering. So I've got some ideas of furthering my studies. *(Alice Springs, studying for undergraduate degree).*

Some young Indigenous males aspired to be the first in their family to attend university, allowing them to share their skills and perspectives with the others:

> University was the only opportunity for me to showcase my skills in the world. I am the first person in my family go to university, so that also makes it more valuable, I would say. *(Canberra, studying for undergraduate degree).*

Mystification of Higher Education

A few participants developed a mystified view of higher education during high school, viewing it as an imposing system that they perceived to be more difficult to navigate than TAFE:

> There was one stage where I wanted to be an audio engineer, because I was into music and all that type of stuff. So, I did think about uni, but I saw it as like this massive, grand thing, compared to TAFE in a sense — for some reason. It's just the way that high schools make it seem. *(Perth, studying for undergraduate degree).*

Discussing the processes of university, particularly flexible study structures, demystified them, potentially opening up pathways for other Indigenous males:

> I'm like, "Well I've got this one-hour class here, and I can watch this lecture whenever I want." And they're [high school students] wowed by that, that that's all I have to do. It sort of lowers that barrier to entry and sort of makes them think about how they could fit that into their life. *(Bendigo, studying for undergraduate degree).*

Influence of Family and Community Education Values

Community and education were explicitly linked in a cycle where shared community, family and individual values compelled young Indigenous males to seek a higher education qualification, allowing them to materially invest in, and contribute back to, their communities. Education values were passed down intergenerationally through family members who had engaged in university in some way, whether through the completion of a degree or through past participation.

> I think having my dad, my Indigenous side, my dad, having an education was a big part [of the motivation to attend university] for me. He always strived to want me to be able to do better than he did. As a father, I guess, you always want to push — you want your kids to grow up and become a better person, or something like that. Yeah, I think my dad having an education, and his mum, and then his nanna having an education *(Alice Springs, studying for undergraduate degree).*
>
> One of the things that was probably driving me to achieve in those first few years at uni was, having this dream of going back to where I grew up or where my mother and father grew up to help address some of the issues out there, and playing more of a medical role in that in being a doctor in these rural and regional communities. So that was something that I sort of used to feel my drive at that point, to be in a position where I could then help people out there. *(Brisbane, studying for Masters degree).*

Students attributed their motivation toward higher education to many community and family members who played an important role in their journey. This highlights how the cumulative advice from multiple people, with diverse expertise, is critical to initiate and sustain a journey into and through higher education:

> Connect with your mentors, and the people that are there to support you. And if you're ever stuck, always ask questions. *(Perth, studying for undergraduate degree).*
>
> When the family started coming to the plays and things, what I was capable of, they were like, okay. So, that was also support, inviting my grandparents to see that it wasn't all just talk, it wasn't all just this. *(Perth, studying for undergraduate degree).*

Increased Life and Career Opportunities

Participants acknowledged the need to acquire diverse skill sets through their qualification, to protect against job losses and shortages, particularly amidst COVID-19.

> It [higher education] allows you to be competitive in this economic market. For example, my skills are transferrable to almost every industry, so it'll allow me to expand and be able to work in a bunch of different areas. *(Canberra, studying for undergraduate degree).*
>
> I think now looking at it, I think everyone should go to uni. Especially in the current climate, there's job loss going around everywhere. There are people with law degrees trying to get jobs at Target. You know what I mean? You need some sort of paper, everything is about paper these days. Like it's good that you have 20 years of experience, but if you have a degree, like it puts you above the rest kind of thing. *(Brisbane, studying for undergraduate degree).*

Overall, the participants tended to favour degrees that had clear vocational pathways and an explicit career trajectory, with high levels of employability.

> I picked it [degree] because I see that as a straight line to a career. Like, I study O.T. [Occupational Therapy], I can become an O.T. Whereas people that study sport science, or stuff like that, there's not a – I didn't want to get my degree, and then struggle to find a job. Or still be in the dark on what I want to do exactly. *(Melbourne, studying for undergraduate degree).*

Many formed career aspirations during their higher education studies through an understanding of the various skill required to succeed within their chosen field. It was perceived that professional progression could be stymied without a qualification or specialised skillsets. Consequently, some students expected increased freedom and flexibility after completing their degree:

> I haven't experienced any computer science projects yet, but what I would know is just by looking at the student handbooks is that – so for one, my career helps me because I'm able to pick specific projects to help me for those units, and then also university would help me in understanding the required techniques or algorithms that the industry uses that enable me to sort of spread my horizons I guess *(Perth, studying for undergraduate degree).*

Representation of Indigenous Perspectives and Methods of Knowledge Translation

Indigenous content is often covered in Australian university and high school courses, however, the quality of the content can be lacking, and the pedagogic practices used may be inappropriate (Carter et al., 2018). Poor instruction around Indigenous content is disrespectful toward Indigenous people as the traditional custodians of their epistemologies, traditions, and worldviews, and misinterpreting Indigenous knowledge risks perpetuating negative stereotypes. Some of the males we spoke with highlighted how Australian universities foregrounded a Western approach to knowledge:

> It's the difference between making Indigenous content as the way of embedding it is just making it the content. So like for science, we're just going to learn about how they used to make an axe, rather than actually embedding ways of knowing, like learning, like using learning circles or different oral histories or oral transmission, those kinds of things, rather than just, okay, we're going to learn about this. And it's still done in a very Western way. *(Brisbane, studying for undergraduate degree).*
>
> It felt wrong because it was coming from a Western understanding of getting Indigenous knowledge, which is wrong. Like flat out wrong. Like it's not how you teach. If you're going to embed it, then you've got to come from an Indigenous standpoint. *(Brisbane, studying for undergraduate degree).*

These insights are consistent with previous research which emphasises how education systems place multiple constraints on Indigenous people participating and achieving in higher education and how the presentation of knowledge and failure to incorporate Indigenous knowledges appropriately can lead to feelings of alienation or a loss of connection (Behrendt et al., 2012; Frawley Smith & Larkin, 2015; Smith et al., 2017; Wood et al., 2019).

Interest in the topic/field.

When discussing the motivations to attend university, the males we spoke with often expressed conflicting feelings about pursuing a topic of interest or studying explicitly for financial purposes. This finding supports existing literature highlighting self-efficacy as a powerful driver of success in higher education among Indigenous Australians (Frawley et al., 2017b). Furthermore, the short-term financial hardships associated with studying were often balanced against the longer-term gains of a personally, professionally, and financially fulfilling career:

> If I had to give a broad sort of answer it would be, to definitely do something that you're interested in. And you're passionate about don't just do it for the money or because you're expected to do it... There are going to be a few years there where it's going to be a bit of a struggle, but if you're doing something you're passionate about then that sacrifice is going to pay off in the long run. *(Brisbane, studying for Masters degree).*

Higher Education Engagement and Retention Barriers

Awareness, Promotion, and Understanding of University

Reflecting wider scholarship on barriers for students from equity groups[3] (Oliver et al., 2016), this study identified a lack of promotion or information available to Indigenous males as being a common barrier inhibiting their engagement in a university course:

> There wasn't much information out there as well, to think that university isn't just this big, grand thing – and I can do it, I just need to put my mind to it. (*Perth, studying for undergraduate degree).*
>
> I had no idea until I even signed up what university structure really was. So I think bridging that gap and just getting the knowledge there that university isn't as hard. *(Bendigo, studying for undergraduate degree).*

Adjustments to Different Environments and Worldviews

The males often viewed university as a foreign place, highlighting that Western institutions often expect students to move interstate to access courses, drawing them away from their family and country:

> So I started at the University of Newcastle. And it was too far. I was downtown and I was the only one. Like there was no family around me, so I ended up moving to UQ because most [family] are from around Brisbane and close to Brisbane, so a couple of hours out of Brisbane so those were the factors for me to move to Brisbane was definitely being close to home. *(Brisbane, studying for undergraduate degree).*
>
> I probably get most of my thoughts from… growing up in the Territory, away, in the area where a lot of people, say from Victoria, New South Wales, just haven't experienced that other world that we are from. I use another world sort of analogy quite a lot, because it is significantly different. I think it's because a lot of the parents aren't educated from the beginning. Some of the kids might not even know what university is, to be honest. *(Alice Springs, studying for undergraduate degree).*

They often expressed a sense of disconnection from the 'host' city, the universities, and their peers, leading to feelings of isolation and a longing for home.

> I've always found that university can be a pretty lonely place coming from high school where there's a lot of connection every single day. And I think it's, yeah real important to keep bringing the community together. *(Bendigo, studying for undergraduate degree).*

In some instances, the men perceived larger cities as daunting, foreign, and distant places to live and study making interstate transitions to attend university even more difficult:

> Coming from a town that's only got 20-odd thousand people, then coming to uni and there's people everywhere. Bendigo's got 100-odd thousand people. I drove up, so I was nervous

---

[3] 'Equity groups' refer to students from low socio-economic backgrounds, non-English speaking backgrounds, rural and remote regions and Indigenous identified students (https://www.dese.gov.au/higher-education-statistics/resources/2017-section-11-equity-groups)

from the start, trying to drive, and traffic I wasn't used to and that sort of stuff, trying to get in there. *(Alice Springs, studying for undergraduate degree).*

These findings suggest there is a great need for universities to be welcoming and culturally safe spaces that embed Indigenous focused content within courses and grow Indigenous support staff based on campus (Buckskin & Tranthim-Fryer, 2018; Pechenkina et al., 2011; Robertson et al., 2021; Smith & Robertson, 2020).

Academic Preparation and Motivation Through School

Many of the young males reported that their high school teachers motivated them to engage with higher education by providing advice and encouragement:

> There was definitely a teacher at the school, *name redacted*, who ran this tutoring program for Aboriginal and Torres Strait [Islander] only students, at the school. And he was someone who was very motivating for me and gave me a lot of good advice and really encouraged me to pursue that and to do as well as I could in school. So I feel like he was a very key influence over me going down that direction to university. *(Brisbane, studying for Masters degree).*

Some reported feeling ill-prepared for university due to poor literacy and numeracy skill development through school, which created low academic achievement expectations and a healthy scepticism about what the education system offered at a personal level:

> You know it's probably the big two, numeracy and literacy. The minute that you can't do one of those things you're seen as dumb and then you're cast out very early on, and then it's almost a fight back just to get to baseline where everyone else is in making that jump to university. Because most people start with they can choose to go to university or TAFE very early on. It's their choice to make. And I think for us, we are sort of – you're going to TAFE if you want to do something and you need to make that next leap and fight and claw to get to university. *(Bendigo, studying for undergraduate degree).*
>
> A lot of them [Indigenous males] just perceive themselves as not being smart enough as well, when you talk to them at school. And that's the thing, you are smart enough to be able to go to uni. Everyone can go to uni, and there's the support for you when you need it. *(Alice Springs, studying for undergraduate degree).*

These findings highlight the intertwined relationship between academic skills and self-efficacy as important drivers of university engagement despite numerous, well documented challenges for Indigenous males to engage in higher education (Day et al., 2015).

Financial Constraints

Indigenous males often hold the 'breadwinner' role in their families, which places pressure upon them to get a job and provide for their families (Reilly & Rees, 2018). This cultural expectation can make it challenging for young Indigenous men to invest in longer-term education pathways. Those we spoke with reflected on this tension:

Aboriginal males, when they leave school, having the need to just get a job straight away to start in and earn money. That may have came from backgrounds that were lower sort of socio-economic and they could understand the value in having money and being able to earn it from an early age. *(Brisbane, studying for master's degree).*

Financial instability adversely affected many of the Indigenous males during their studies, particularly the short-term financial risks of continuing study caused by the stress of covering rent and other household expenses, although this was less evident among young Indigenous males when compared to their older counterparts.

Trying to be independent in regards to having a gym membership, going to the gym, having enough money for food so that I can have a routine and that I can make my own meals and not eat garbage so that it effects the way my brain functions, just really simple things like that. They can be challenging sometimes as well *(Canberra, studying for undergraduate degree).*

There was a salient risk of incurring a lifelong debt for participants, a significant disincentive to commencing or continuing study:

So many employers from all these different industries want Indigenous people, but the thing stopping them [young Indigenous people] now is literally just the HECS debt and the future fees that they may have to come. And that could be the difference of going to university or not going to university. *(Perth, studying for undergraduate degree).*

Participants that moved interstate to attend university often could not afford to return home to be closer to family and Country. The importance of home was essential, especially when considered as a retreat from the foreign and demanding atmosphere of university:

When I left college and I had to go and find my own place. I didn't have the money to fly home as regularly as I could. Those times I definitely struggled a lot more. *(Brisbane, studying for undergraduate degree).*

Factors Influencing Study Engagement and Success

Online Learning

Several participants had successfully adapted to online learning during COVID-19 lockdowns reporting positive benefits from working at home with no disruptions to coursework:

I do work as a programmer, so most of the stuff I do anyways I can work from home, so units like chemistry and the rest, that didn't impact me. I actually thrived in that sort of situation. *(Perth, studying for undergraduate degree).*

Some found it challenging to complete coursework online in some fields, needing in-person assistance from academic staff.

I mean, one of the personal impacts for myself was probably just having to drop my math unit. I can't do math online. It just doesn't work out for me. I've always needed a tutor to sit beside me and just show me sort of what to do, the different ways to do it. *(Perth, studying for undergraduate degree).*

COVID-19 Disruptions to Study

Although several participants described the benefits of online learning during COVID-19, others were aware of hardships experienced by their classmates that remained on campus:

> Hearing the stories from other people that stayed here on campus, or were in the lockdowns in metropolitan, it was a lot different and a lot tougher. *(Alice Springs, studying for undergraduate degree).*

Financial Support and the Importance of Scholarships

In many instances, financial assistance (e.g., scholarships) from universities and other organisations funded participants education, and covered other personal expenses (e.g., renting accommodation), as they often had little financial support from their families. Some Indigenous males may have gone into debt without a scholarship, which created immense stress and academic disengagement. Socioeconomic disadvantage can often exclude Indigenous males from higher education as they need to earn and support their families, often from a young age.

> I don't have any financial support from family at all. So if I wasn't able to afford it myself, I couldn't do it. At that particular time, my income versus my rent was – I was in a deficit every single week, so I never got to a surplus. As a result, it just put too much strain on me, I couldn't focus on uni, and I dropped out. This time round, I was fortunate enough to receive a scholarship. That's one of the big reasons I came to Canberra. I got the scholarship, and that helped me, confidence-wise, to alleviate any of the financial strains I knew I was going to encounter. *(Canberra, studying for undergraduate degree).*

> Aboriginal males, when they leave school, having the need to just get a job straight away to start in and earn money. That may have come from backgrounds that were lower sort of socio-economic and they could understand the value in having money and being able to earn it from an early age. *(Brisbane, studying for Masters degree).*

Indigenous Support Units at Universities

The importance of the Indigenous Support Units at universities was clearly highlighted as beneficial by participants. The Units contributed to participants' increased access to universities as well as success, retention, completion, and satisfaction within a university environment. This support was very well-regarded by participants, particularly in the context of an otherwise often unwelcoming campus and long bouts of isolation, exacerbated by travel. Support officers within study units often build community networks that support the promotion of university courses and the recruitment of Indigenous males. These staff often undertake this role outside of their primary work supporting existing students.

> So there was a lot of support from the Jimbeyer unit from the get-go, which helped significantly. Yeah, went to accommodation services, got my room key, all that sort of stuff, and

went to the Hillside Apartments, which is where I'm staying. Yeah, it was good. The people in there that was already living there from the start, were very friendly, very good, so I got along really well. *(Alice Springs, studying for undergraduate degree).*

No, I really appreciate the Ngunnawal Centre's help, especially in my first year, I kind of had no idea what I was doing at Uni a bit. The Ngunnawal Centre was a good place to go for focus and come to grasps, and it was a good place to study and hang out when I had free periods or free time. *(Canberra, studying for undergraduate degree).*

Routines and Schedules

University structures and routines supported participants to attend classes and meet deadlines. Study plans were essential in allowing students the flexibility to meet their deadlines:

You get into your routine, you get your patterns, and it's the same with school. You've got your timetable, pretty much your classes are here, here and here. You've got your homework to do, yeah, it's just a bigger version of school, basically, I found. Putting it in that perspective helped me a lot. *(Alice Springs, studying for undergraduate degree).*

One of the biggest supportive mechanisms that's allowed me to overcome this to the point where I have is the RAP [Reconciliation Action Plan], the RAP plan that was put in place by the university that allowed me to negotiate timelines for my assignments. That's been massive, because there has been a lot of times when the days would arise that an assignment was due and I'd partially completed it, but I'd needed a mental health day because I would trigger, for example. And so, that was immensely helpful. *(Canberra, studying for undergraduate degree).*

However, in some instances the lack of formal schedules was challenging for students transitioning to higher education who were not used to creating and managing their own routines:

I do find it hard to sit down and study, I do get – I procrastinate a lot, but I think I also — I think it's been solely up to me to make my own study schedule. So, there's been no real support to show me skills in life to sit down and just get things done. It's just been for me – it's been up to me to sort of just go round and try things. *(Canberra, studying for undergraduate degree).*

While some Indigenous males sought out formal support and some did not, previous research has documented how males – especially males from non-traditional or first-in-family backgrounds – can be reluctant to seek support (Alexander, 2017; O'Shea et al., 2017; Stahl, 2021).

Mindset and Self-Efficacy

Mindset and self-efficacy played a notable role in participants' study persistence. Some participants commenced courses with a clear focus and high motivation levels, while some developed it during their courses, often using perceived failures to strengthen their mindset, motivation and discipline:

I think a challenge for me was getting out of that mindset, where I was like, "Oh I'm doing well." doing the bare minimum. I wasn't really learning as much as I could from the subject. Trying to force myself out of that habit, and actively involve myself. *(Melbourne, studying for undergraduate degree).*

It wasn't until I failed twice, that my brain rewired itself to become so disciplined, that no matter what I do, I'm going to complete it. *(Perth, studying for undergraduate degree).*

Discussion: Implications for Policy and Practice

Promotion of Programs and Role Models

This study highlights the importance of sharing family and community experiences of university that may inspire young Indigenous males to begin and persist with their studies. Participants identified a need to demystify higher education, its institutions and study structures, often citing role models and course marketing as essential reference points to clarify concerns. Many of the participants in this study identified themselves as community role models, which motivated them to share their journeys to and through university, often hoping that it would inspire other young males to engage in higher education. Therefore, it is recommended that universities, and the bridging courses they offer, highlight Indigenous community members, current students and alumni (particularly males) as role models, sharing their education stories in resources and promotional campaigns to attract and retain Indigenous males in higher education. Focusing the advertising on tangible, clear course pathway options and outcomes supports our findings and existing literature focusing on the need to increase Indigenous students' engagement with higher education (Rochecouste et al., 2017). Ideally, these resources and campaigns should be promoted through high schools, vocational education training settings, sports clubs, and community networks, to illuminate education and career pathways for potential students at critical life junctures. Collaborative relationships and articulation agreements between VET and higher education will be critical in encouraging greater uptake of university-level studies by Indigenous males. Indigenous support centres within VET and HE could be important conduits for promotion.

Echoing previous research on indigenous masculinities in Australian higher education (Stahl et al., 2020), participants identified that opportunities to influence change in their communities motivated them to enrol and participate in university. Indigenous students were more likely to believe that their qualifications would improve welfare in their community compared to their non-Indigenous peers (Asmar et al., 2015). To effectively promote higher education qualifications to Indigenous males, it is useful to highlight the potential for improved health, education, and welfare outcomes for Indigenous people. This will have a greater impact than promoting prospective financial gain, which participants reported as being less influential. This seems particularly relevant for health and community service sectors, where Indigenous males have historically been under-represented.

Online Courses

A major barrier for Indigenous males to study was the requirement to relocate, leave family and community, and adapt to a worldview and environment that many found foreign and, in some instances, culturally unsafe. Higher education institutions seek to bring students into what is predominantly a Western domain, a process that is often unsettling and creates a sense of disconnection and loneliness.

For the participants of the study, the rise of online courses during COVID-19 had the capacity to improve work-life balance with often minimal disruption to courses. Increased offerings of online courses could allow students in remote locations to stay in their community and Country with family, improving social and emotional wellbeing, potentially reducing the financial burden of relocating or renting, and the conflict of trading family and community responsibilities for university (Pollard, 2018; Shalley et al., 2019). Additional investment and support to ensure internet connectivity is essential and would also be required (Pollard, 2018).

Regional study hubs provide material and academic supports for students in remote places (Napthine et al., 2018). Government grants for libraries and community centres in remote locations could expand the network of study hubs and provide computers, and study materials designed to increase higher education awareness, computer literacy and ultimately participation in online university courses (Hossain et al., 2008; Pollard, 2018). Universities could offer in-kind contributions to these communal spaces, providing free classes, equipment, and resources to simultaneously build relationships while improving higher education awareness and engagement (Hossain et al., 2008; Pollard, 2018). Similarly, scholarships to support IT infrastructure, such as the purchase of laptops and internet access, would also be beneficial (Pollard, 2018). Investments in adult English language and literacy is also advisable to maximise the benefit of such investments (Shalley et al., 2019).

Further research is needed to fully understand Indigenous males' perceptions of online learning as Australian undergraduate students reported adverse mental health and wellbeing impacts stemming from online courses (Dodd et al., 2021). Further research with Indigenous males examining the potential positive mental health and wellbeing benefits of remaining connected to Country, community, and family through the provision of online education and support options, and how these might offset feelings of disconnection and isolation experienced by an inability to engage in face-to-face learning, is also required. Some higher education courses are not well suited to online learning, so face-to-face options may still be preferred in many cases (Mullen et al., 2021; Seymour-Walsh et al., 2020). Providing Indigenous mentors and study programs to support students both on-campus and online would help them to develop schedules and advocate for flexible deadlines. Self-efficacy must be at the forefront of pedagogic approaches to support student wellbeing and engagement (Frawley et al., 2017a, b, c; Wilson et al., 2019). As highlighted by participants, university is a fast-changing environment intensified by COVID-19 and the development of online courses, so it is important that students develop self-efficacy to sustain study engagement and wellbeing.

Indigenous Study Units and Cultural Spaces on Campus

Some students preferred to stay on campus, identifying adverse effects from online study while promoting the benefits of Indigenous study units, which served multiple roles as places to foster friendships and share knowledge and culture. These spaces provide access to social, cultural, accommodation, study, and financial support, all of which are key social and cultural determinants of health (Islam, 2019). Indigenous study units serve a role similar to gathering or meeting places in community settings which are safe spaces to share and practice language and culture, reducing feelings of alienation and disconnection (Kingsley et al., 2018). It will be important to seek further advice from a range of geographically, culturally, and linguistically diverse Indigenous males to provide appropriate staff, resources, and languages to support the integration and expansion of these study units.

We suggest that having Indigenous-identified support staff to improve cultural competence at universities is urgently needed. In this instance, cultural competence refers to those who are from Indigenous cultures and thus can understand and interpret them (Frawley et al., 2020). It is important to employ Indigenous staff to promote a shared understanding and worldview with students and serve as role models who can provide study assistance. When combined with Indigenous study units, these staff may support dual improvements in student health, well-being, and educational outcomes.

A key challenge to maximising the impact of Indigenous centres within universities is the reluctance of many institutions to contribute funding to their work beyond the Commonwealth Government's contribution through the Indigenous Student Success Program (ISSP) (Department of the Prime Minister and Cabinet, 2018). Supplementary funding to support this work is often the sole source of funds for the recruitment, retention, and success of Indigenous students (Buckskin & Tranthim-Fryer, 2018; Hearn & Kenna, 2020). This concern is highlighted by the Commonwealth Government's requirement for universities to now report funding committed to Indigenous student success that extends beyond this specialist grant scheme (Department of the Prime Minister and Cabinet, 2018). The new Indigenous, Regional, Low-SES Attainment Fund (IRSLAF) provides further resources for universities to attract and retain Indigenous students. However, it remains vital for universities to invest their own core funding to make progress towards closing educational attainment gaps between Indigenous and non-Indigenous students.

Financial Support

For Indigenous males experiencing cumulative equity impacts, such as remoteness and lower socio-economic status, scholarships for course fees and living expenses allow access to education (Barney, 2013). Financial challenges are the most prominent reason Indigenous students considered leaving their program (at almost twice the rate of non-Indigenous peers) (Asmar et al., 2015). The men who took part in this study expressed gratitude for scholarships focused on tuition fees, accommodation, and IT support. We recommend that universities continue expanding upon forms of financial assistance that will encourage and sustain more Indigenous students to pursue their higher education aspirations. This is particularly important for students from rural and more remote settings (Pollard, 2018).

Conclusion

This chapter has provided a holistic view of strategies to increase Indigenous males' participation and achievement in higher education. We have identified and discussed ways to remove barriers to participation and sustain students' engagement in proactive ways. We have deliberately adopted a cultural and social determinants of health lens in viewing our findings as consistent with the holistic understandings of health and wellbeing promoted by national Aboriginal and Torres Strait Islander policies and frameworks. In doing so, we have identified health promotion strategies that will: (1) increase Indigenous males' participation and achievement in higher education; (2) foster cultural safety and responsiveness; and (3) enhance financial security. We encourage Australian universities to adopt these strategies to enhance the lives of Indigenous males, and ultimately those of their families and the communities in which they live.

References

Alexander, P. (2017). Coming of age through the recession: High school imaginings of post-recession futures in new York City. In G. Stahl, J. Nelson, & D. O. Wallace (Eds.), *Masculinity and aspiration in the era of neoliberal education: International perspectives* (pp. 89–108). Routledge.

Asmar, C., Page, S., & Radloff, A. (2015). Exploring anomalies in indigenous student engagement: Findings from a national Australian survey of undergraduates. *Higher Education Research and Development, 34*(1), 15–29. https://doi.org/10.1080/07294360.2014.934334

Australian Indigenous HealthInfoNet. (2018). *Overview of aboriginal and Torres Strait islander health status, 2017*. Australian Indigenous HealthInfoNet.

Australian Institute of Health and Welfare. (2012). *The health of Australia's males: A focus on five population groups. Cat. No. PHE160*. Australian Government.

Barney, K. (2013). "taking your mob with you": Giving voice to the experiences of indigenous Australian postgraduate students. *Higher Education Research and Development, 32*(4), 515–528. https://doi.org/10.1080/07294360.2012.696186

Behrendt, L., Larkin, S., Griew, R., & Kelly, P. (2012). *Review of higher education access and outcomes for aboriginal and Torres Strait islander people: Final report*. Australian Government.

Buckskin, P., & Tranthim-Fryer, M. (2018). *Accelerating indigenous higher education: Consultation paper*. National Aboriginal and Torres Strait Islander Higher Education Consortium.

Carter, J., Hollinsworth, D., Raciti, M., & Gilbey, K. (2018). Academic 'place-making': Fostering attachment, belonging and identity for indigenous students in Australian universities. *Teaching in Higher Education, 23*(2), 243–260. https://doi.org/10.1080/13562517.2017.1379485

Day, A., Nakata, V., Nakata, M., & Martin, G. (2015). Indigenous students' persistence in higher education in Australia: Contextualising models of change from psychology to understand and aid students' practices at a cultural interface. *Higher Education Research and Development, 34*(3), 501–512. https://doi.org/10.1080/07294360.2014.973379

Department of Education, Skills and Employment. (2020). *Selected higher education statistics – 2019 student data*. Australia.

Department of Health. (2019). *National Men's health strategy 2020–2030*. Commonwealth of Australia.

Department of the Prime Minister and Cabinet. (2018). ISSP Post-Implementation Review 2018. https://www.niaa.gov.au/sites/default/files/publications/ISSP-review-discussion-paper-2018.pdf

Dodd, R. H., Dadaczynski, K., Okan, O., McCaffery, K. J., & Pickles, K. (2021). Psychological Well-being and academic experience of university students in Australia during COVID-19. *International Journal of Environmental Research and Public Health, 18*(3), 866. https://doi.org/10.3390/IJERPH18030866

Frawley Smith, J., & Larkin, S. (2015). Beyond Bradley and Behrendt: Building a stronger evidence-base about indigenous pathways and transitions into higher education. *Learning Communities: International Journal of Learning in Social Contexts, 17*, 8–11.

Frawley, O., Olcay, R., & Smith, J. (2017a). *Indigenous achievement in higher education and the role of self-efficacy: Rippling stories of success*. National Centre for Student Equity in Higher Education.

Frawley, J., Ober, R., Olcay, M., & Smith, J. A. (2017b). Indigenous achievement in higher education and the role of self-efficacy: Rippling stories of success. In *National Centre for student equity in higher education (NCSEHE)*. Curtin University.

Frawley, J., Smith, J., & Larkin, S. (2017c). From policy to practice in higher education: Cross-cutting issues in indigenous pathways, transition and participation. In J. Frawley, S. Larkin, & J. Smith (Eds.), *Indigenous pathways, transitions and participation in higher education: From policy to practice*. Springer.

Frawley, J., Russell, G., & Sherwood, J. (2020). *Cultural competence and the higher education sector*. Springer.

Gupta, H., Smith, J., Fleay, J., Lesiter, C. P. B., & Canuto, K. (2021). Understanding the nexus between alcohol consumption, social and emotional wellbeing, and higher education outcomes among Aboriginal and Torres Strait islander males in Australia. *International Journal of Men's Social and Community Health, 4*(1), e28–e37. https://doi.org/10.22374/ijmsch.v4i1.52

Hearn, S., & Kenna, L. (2020). Spending for success: Identifying "what works?" for indigenous student outcomes in Australian universities. *Australian Journal of Indigenous Education., 50*, 237–246. https://doi.org/10.1017/jie.2020.27

Hossain, D., Gorman, D., Williams-Mozely, J., & Garvey, D. (2008). Bridging the gap: Identifying needs and aspirations of indigenous students to their entry into university. *Australian Journal of Indigenous Education, 37*(1), 9–17. https://doi.org/10.1017/S1326011100016045

Islam, M. M. (2019). Social determinants of health and related inequalities: Confusion and implications. *Frontiers in public health, 7*:11 (February), 11–14. https://doi.org/10.3389/fpubh.2019.00011

Kingsley, J., Munro-Harrison, E., Jenkins, A., & Thorpe, A. (2018). "Here we are part of a living culture": Understanding the cultural determinants of health in aboriginal gathering places in Victoria, Australia. *Health & Place, 54*, 210–220. https://doi.org/10.1016/J.HEALTHPLACE.2018.10.001

Lovett, R., Lee, V., Kukutai, T., Cormack, D., Rainie, S. C., & Walker, J. (2019). *Good data practices for indigenous data sovereignty and governance, good data* (pp. 26–36). Institute of Network Cultures.

Mullen, C., Pettigrew, J., Cronin, A., Rylands, L., & Shearman, D. (2021). Mathematics is different: Student and tutor perspectives from Ireland and Australia on online support during COVID-19. *Teaching Mathematics and its Applications: An International Journal of the IMA, 40*(4), 332–355. https://doi.org/10.1093/TEAMAT/HRAB014

Napthine, D., Lee, P., Graham, C., & Wills, M. (2018). National regional, rural and remote education strategy: Final report. In: *Department of Education and Training.* https://www.education.gov.au/national-regional-rural-and-remote-education-strategy

O'Shea, S., May, J., Stone, C., & Delahunty, J. (2017). First-in-family students, university experience and family life: Motivations, transitions and participation. *London: Palgrave Macmillan.* https://doi.org/10.1057/978-1-137-58284-3

Oliver, R., Grote, E., Rochecouste, J., & Dann, T. (2016). Indigenous student perspectives on support and impediments at university. *Australian Journal of Indigenous Education, 45*(1), 23–35. https://doi.org/10.1017/JIE.2015.16

Pechenkina, E., Kowal, E., & Paradies, Y. (2011). Indigenous Australian students' participation rates in higher education: Exploring the role of universities. *Australian Journal of Indigenous Education, 40*(2011), 59–68. https://doi.org/10.1375/ajie.40.59

Pollard, L. (2018). *Remote student university success: An analysis of policy and practice. An equity fellowship report prepared for the National Centre for student equity in higher education.* Curtin University and the University of Western Australia.

Reilly, L., & Rees, S. (2018). Fatherhood in Australian aboriginal and Torres Strait islander communities: An examination of barriers and opportunities to strengthen the male parenting role. *American Journal of Men's Health, 12*(2), 420–430. https://doi.org/10.1177/1557988317735928

Robertson, K., Smith, J., & Larkin, S. (2021). Improving higher education success for Australian indigenous peoples. In N. Harrison & G. Atherton (Eds.), *Marginalised communities in higher education: Disadvantage, mobility and indigeneity.* Routledge.

Rochecouste, J., Oliver, R., Bennell, D., Anderson, R., Cooper, I., & Forrest, S. (2017). Teaching Australian aboriginal higher education students: What should universities do? *Studies in Higher Education, 42*(11), 2080–2098. https://doi.org/10.1080/03075079.2015.1134474

Seymour-Walsh, A. E., Bell, A., Weber, A., & Smith, T. (2020). Adapting to a new reality: COVID-19 coronavirus and online education in the health professions. *Rural and Remote Health, 20*(2), 6000. https://doi.org/10.22605/rrh6000

Shalley, F., Smith, J., Wood, D., Fredericks, B., & Robertson, K. (2019). *Understanding completion rates of indigenous higher education students from two regional universities: A cohort analysis.* National Centre for Student Equity in Higher Education.

Shankar, J., Ip, E., Khalema, E., Couture, J., Tan, S., Zulla, R. T., & Lam, G. (2013). Education as a social determinant of health: Issues facing indigenous and visible minority students in post-secondary education in Western Canada. *International Journal of Environmental Research and Public Health, 10*(9), 3908–3929. https://doi.org/10.3390/IJERPH10093908

Smith, J. (2018). A National Men's health strategy in Australia: Tips for implementation. *International Journal of Men's Social and Community Health, 1*(1), e15–e21.

Smith, J., & Robertson, K. (2020). Evaluating cultural competence in indigenous higher education contexts in Australia: A challenge for change. In J. Frawley, G. Russell, & J. Sherwood (Eds.), *Cultural competence and the higher education section: Australian perspectives, policies, and practice* (pp. 117–136). Springer.

Smith, J., Frawley, J., Pechenkina, E., Ludwig, W., Robertson, C., Gunstone, A., & Larkin, S. (2017). *Identifying strategies for promoting VET to higher education transitions for indigenous learners.* National Centre for Student Equity in Higher Education.

Smith, J., Bullot, M., Kerr, V., Yibarbuk, D., Olcay, M., & Shalley, F. (2018). Maintaining connection to family, culture and community: Implications for remote Aboriginal and Torres Strait Islander pathways into higher education. *Rural Society, 27*(2), 108–124.

Smith, J., Drummond, M., Adams, M., Bonson, J., & Christie, B. (2019). Understanding inequities in men's health in Australia. In D. Griffith, M. Bruce, & R. Thorpe (Eds.), *Men's health equity: A handbook* (pp. 499–511). Routledge.

Smith, J., Merlino, A., Christie, B., Adams, M., Bonson, J., Osborne, R., Judd, B., Drummond, M., Aanundsen, D., & Fleay, J. (2020). 'Dudes are meant to be tough as nails': The complex nexus between masculinities, cultural and health literacy from the perspective of young aboriginal and Torres Strait islander males — Implications for policy and practice. *American Journal of Men's Health, 14*(3), 1–17.

Smith, J. A., Gupta, H., Moore, S., Fleay, J., Stahl, G., Uink, B., Harvey, A., Radoll, P., Hill, B., Bennett, R., Vigona, J., & Merlino, A. (2022). *Higher education aspirations, participation, and achievement of Australian indigenous males. Report prepared for the National Centre for student equity in higher education.* Curtin University.

Stahl, G. (2021). *Working-class masculinities in Australian higher education: Policies, pathways and Progress.* Routledge.

Stahl, G., McDonald, S., & Stokes, J. (2020). 'I see myself as undeveloped': Supporting indigenous first-in-family males in the transition to higher education. *Higher Education Research & Development, 39*(7), 1488–1501. https://doi.org/10.1080/07294360.2020.1728521

Lowitja Institute. (2014). *Cultural wounds require cultural medicine: Background paper.* Cultural determinants roundtable, Melbourne, 26 November 2014. https://www.lowitja.org.au/content/Document/PDF/Cultural-Determinants-Roundtable-Background-Paper.pdf

Tomaszewski, W., Kubler, M., Perales, P., Western, M., Ramino, T., & Xiang, N. (2018). *Review of identified equity groups.* Institute for Social Science Research.

Walter, M., & Suina, M. (2019). Indigenous data, indigenous methodologies and indigenous data sovereignty. *International Journal of Social Research Methodology, 22*(3), 233–243.

Wilson, B., Abbott, T., Quinn, S. J., Guenther, J., McRae-Williams, E., & Cairney, S. (2019). Empowerment is the basis for improving education and employment outcomes for aboriginal people in remote Australia. *The Australian Journal of Indigenous Education, 48*(2), 153–161. https://doi.org/10.1017/JIE.2018.2

Wood, D., Fredericks, B., Smith, J., Watkin-Lui, F., Larkin, S., Gruppetta, M., & Rigney, L. I. (2019). *Addressing the gap between policy and implementation: Strategies for improving the educational outcomes of indigenous students. Final report prepared for the Office of Learning and Teaching.* National Centre for Student Equity in Higher Education.

Chapter 9
Applying Indigenous Data Sovereignty Principles to Research with Young Indigenous Males: Lessons for Health Promotion from a Higher Education Project in Australia

Himanshu Gupta, James A. Smith, Garth Stahl, Andrew Harvey, Braden Hill, and Jesse J. Fleay

Introduction and Background

Aboriginal and Torres Strait Islander people (respectfully Indigenous hereon) face multiple challenges when striving to participate and achieve in higher education (Behrendt et al., 2012; Frawley et al., 2015; Frawley et al., 2017; Wood et al., 2019). In Australia, men are under-represented in higher education across all equity groups, except for women in non-traditional areas (Bradley et al., 2008; Tomaszewski et al.,

H. Gupta · J. A. Smith (✉)
Freemasons Centre for Male Health and Wellbeing – Northern Territory, Menzies School of Health Research, Charles Darwin University, Darwin, NT, Australia

Rural and Remote Health, College of Medicine and Public Health, Flinders University, Darwin, NT, Australia
e-mail: himanshu.gupta@flinders.edu.au; james.smith@flinders.edu.au

G. Stahl
School of Education, University of Queensland, Brisbane, Australia
e-mail: g.stahl@uq.edu.au

A. Harvey
School of Education, Griffith University, Logan, QLD, Australia
e-mail: Andrew.harvey@griffith.edu.au

B. Hill
Centre of Kurongkurl Katitjin, Edith Cowan University, Mt Lawley, WA, Australia
e-mail: b.hill@ecu.edu.au

J. J. Fleay
School of Education, Curtin University, Bentley, WA, Australia
e-mail: j.fleay@curtin.edu.au

© Menzies School of Health Research, the rights holder, and The Editor(s)
(if applicable) and The Author(s), under exclusive license to Springer Nature
Switzerland AG 2023
J. A. Smith et al. (eds.), *Health Promotion with Adolescent Boys and Young Men of Colour*, https://doi.org/10.1007/978-3-031-22174-3_9

2018). While Indigenous males[1] have reasonable rates of participation in Vocational Education and Training (VET), they are far less likely to engage in university than Indigenous females (Shalley et al., 2019; Smith et al., 2017). This means that Indigenous Australian males face cumulative impacts associated with both gender and race when attempting to pursue higher education (Shalley et al., 2019). Given these barriers, the enrolment, participation, and completion rates of Indigenous males in higher education is a major concern. It is important not to frame this problem as a competition between genders. There are clearly unique and significant challenges that women face, especially those from non-traditional backgrounds, when pursuing education.

As discussed in Chap. 8, the under-representation of Indigenous males in higher education is stark, with very little known about how to increase their participation in higher education. Crucially, there is scant research on why some Indigenous Australian males aspire to higher education and why some do not. Likewise, there is minimal indication that under-representation of Indigenous males has been considered comprehensively within the realms of Indigenous or student equity higher education policy and practice.

In 2012, a review of higher education access and outcomes for Indigenous people provided a clear roadmap for action to achieve parity with non-Indigenous counterparts, which resulted in policy and practice investments across the sector (Behrendt et al., 2012; Frawley et al., 2015). Similarly, a recent Office of Learning and Teaching report identified key enablers for improving educational outcomes for Indigenous higher education across Australia (Wood et al., 2019). For example, a research project funded by the National Centre for Student Equity in Higher Education (NCSEHE) revealed that self-efficacy was a powerful driver of success in higher education among Indigenous Australians (Frawley, Ober, et al., 2017).

Previous research has not offered gender-specific strategies to inform policy and practice improvements for Indigenous males. Given the gendered disparities in higher education access among this cohort, a closer examination of Indigenous male participation and experience at university is needed to address this significant student equity and gender educational gap. Likewise, the higher education sector requires greater understanding of the way university-engaged Indigenous males conceptualise their higher education aspirations, participation, and achievement. Such understandings can help to enhance outreach, engagement and retention activities targeting Indigenous boys and men. Understanding the higher education aspirations of young Indigenous males, and the factors promoting higher education

---

[1] In this study we use the term 'males' rather than 'men'. This is an attempt to acknowledge cultural lore and be inclusive of males who have been through an initiation ceremony and those who have not had the opportunity to do so (Smith et al., 2019; Adams et al., 2021). This is consistent with national policy frameworks relating to, and developed by, Aboriginal and Torres Strait Islander males. The authors recognise that the category 'sex' (male) and 'gender' (men/masculinities) are both important concepts from a dominant Western perspective, and that these terms have different meanings. We maintain that sociological understandings of gender are best understood alongside intersections with age and culture (Merlino et al., 2020; Smith et al., 2020).

participation and achievement of adult Indigenous males, has social and economic benefits that extend beyond the higher education sector. For example, the Australian Government's *National Men's Health Strategy 2020–2030* identifies that education across the life course is a critical social determinant of health (Department of Health, 2019).

Similarly, global evidence suggests that educational interventions aimed at reducing disengagement and attrition from school and higher education can yield wide-ranging benefits for men, particularly young men of colour from both First Nations and African American backgrounds (Australian Indigenous HealthInfoNet, 2018; Australian Institute of Health and Welfare, 2012; Smith et al., 2018; Smith, 2018). In Australia, however, there are currently minimal comparative education-oriented programs tailored for Indigenous males, with the exception of the Clontarf Foundation and a handful of emerging unevaluated programs targeting 'at-risk' or justice-involved Indigenous youth. The limited investment reflects scant research on the unique higher education needs and experiences of this cohort (Gupta et al., 2021; Stahl et al., 2020).

Research examining the relationship between Indigenous males and the higher education system has strong potential to improve policy and practice responses – within the tertiary sector and beyond – and lay the foundation for educational, social, health, and economic improvements. To conduct research ethically, attention must be paid to emerging national and global scholarship regarding Indigenous Data Sovereignty (IDS), and how Indigenous self-determination can be achieved through such responses. In this chapter, we describe how we have applied emerging principles of IDS as we implemented an NCSEHE- funded project entitled "Higher education aspirations, participation and achievement of Australian Indigenous males" (Smith et al., 2022), to help other researchers and practitioners adopt such approaches in future research aiming to improve the health and wellbeing of young Indigenous males. In this chapter, we aim to demonstrate why the historical and philosophical justification for the adoption of IDS is important in this context. Before we describe how we attempted to apply concepts of IDS throughout this project, it is first useful to understand the overarching research approach.

Research Methodology

The project we discuss throughout this chapter involved three distinct but intersecting phases:

Phase 1: Collating success stories of Indigenous male higher education students and alumni.

Indigenous scholarship in Australia has repeatedly emphasised the importance of using strengths-based narratives to inform policy and practice aimed at improving the health and wellbeing of Indigenous peoples (Fogarty et al., 2018). This phase involved individual interviews with Indigenous male higher education students and alumni across five state and territory jurisdictions, namely the Northern Territory, Western Australia, Queensland, Australian Capital Territory and Victoria. Participants were recruited through youth, community, or sporting organisations, and universities with whom the chief investigators already had established relationships.

The interviews, which were video recorded (primarily via Zoom), involved participants talking about the challenges and opportunities they had experienced while participating in, and/or completing, higher education. Interview data was analysed thematically, and the empirical findings have already been presented in Chap. 8.

Phase 2: Identifying success factors to inform policy and practice improvement.

This phase involved most investigators attending a half-day online coding and analysis workshop using Zoom to review the content of the interview transcripts. This involved each researcher talking through the pre-coded transcripts to establish a coding structure that guided subsequent analyses. The primary purpose was to identify success factors specific to Indigenous males, to support future outreach, enable recruitment and retention activities, and strategies planned and implemented by higher education institutions across Australia.

Phase 3: Knowledge translation and impact.

An important aspect of Indigenous-focused research is knowledge translation. To achieve this, we proposed (1) holding a half-day workshop at the conclusion of the study to launch and promote the study findings; (2) releasing the final project report to the public; and (3) discussing the success factors and respective policy and practice strategies identified during Phase 2 with key national stakeholders. We intended for this occur during the World Indigenous Peoples Conference on Education (WIPCE), but COVID-19 has resulted in the conference being rescheduled to 2022, after the project had finished in late 2021.

Each of these phases will be discussed to varying degrees throughout the following discussion on IDS. As these are not necessarily linear or staged processes, there is some overlap.

Adopting Indigenous Data Sovereignty Principles

From a philosophical perspective, the research team was committed to ensuring IDS principles underpinned the way this research was conducted, as per the United Nations Declaration on the Rights of Indigenous Peoples (The United Nations, 2007). There is no simple articulation of IDS in Australia; however, there is plentiful scholarship about Indigenous Australians data needs and rights (Griffiths & Smith, 2020; Walter & Suina, 2019), and why these are important for advancing health promotion practice. As Lovett et al. (2019) argue:

> Good data, including good data governance, are necessary to ensure Indigenous peoples benefit from current and future data practices and to mitigate the potential for continued harm. IDS movements also support broader transformative aims of developing Indigenous-owned and controlled data infrastructures, protocols and community capabilities that lie beyond the reach of nation states and corporations. (Lovett et al., 2019, p. 34)

To address IDS in this project, we used the below principles as described in the Maiam Nayri Wingara Communique (Maiam Nayri Wingara, 2018, p. 2):

In Australia, Indigenous peoples have the right to:

- Exercise control of the data ecosystem including creation, development, stewardship, analysis, dissemination and infrastructure;
- Data that is contextual and disaggregated (available and accessible at individual, community and First Nations levels);
- Data that is relevant and empowers sustainable self-determination and effective self-governance;
- Data structures that are accountable to Indigenous peoples and First Nations; and
- Data that is protective and respects our individual and collective interests.

For this project, we considered a member of the Indigenous community as someone who identifies as an Indigenous person and is interested in the wellbeing of other Indigenous people, specifically Indigenous males. The remainder of the chapter describes how this project has addressed the criteria laid out by Maiam Nayri Wingara in relation to our project.

Exercise Control of the Data Ecosystem Including Creation, Development, Stewardship, Analysis, Dissemination, and Infrastructure

We acknowledged the importance of IDS from the outset of planning for this project (National Centre for Student Equity in Higher Education, 2018). The initial grant proposal was prepared with input from Indigenous scholars from six state and territory jurisdictions across Australia. This included Indigenous senior executives and academics, early career researchers, and graduate student researchers.

Integral to the design of the research was the importance of building respectful research relationships, whereby research benefits and methods were determined by Indigenous stakeholders as the grant proposal was developed. For this reason, we included seven nationally recognised Indigenous scholars/educators as investigators on the research team, in addition to respected non-Indigenous researchers. This process ensured a high level of cultural integrity during the research design process and enhanced the potential for an Indigenist perspective to be adopted throughout all stages of the planning, ethics preparation, fieldwork, analysis, and knowledge dissemination processes. Importantly, one of the project co-leads, an emerging

Indigenous scholar, was mentored by more senior Indigenous and non-Indigenous team members as an explicit Indigenous research capacity building activity.

The research team met monthly throughout the project, ensuring that any challenges or issues emerging in relation to the project could be discussed openly and resolved quickly. This was important for a few different reasons. Several of the investigators were in senior executive roles with demanding workloads, so their engagement in the study ebbed and flowed throughout the course of the project based on other demands on their time, including COVID-19.

One investigator withdrew due to such pressures but remained committed to the intent of the project. Another investigator passed away during the project. Another staff member experienced significant mental health and wellbeing concerns. These circumstances meant that regular communication was critical to keeping the project progressing in a timely and culturally responsive way, and to enhancing relationship development between team members.

Another important example relating to this particular IDS principle was the initial coding process, and subsequent development of a coding framework used throughout the analysis. Due to time constraints, many Indigenous team members were unavailable to assist with the initial coding, which resulted in the draft coding framework being developed by non-Indigenous team members. This was deemed unsatisfactory by both the Indigenous and non-Indigenous team members. Once discussed, the team quickly engaged an Indigenous male team member to review transcripts and amend the coding structure. This ensured a deeper level of Indigenous input into how the data was managed, increasing the cultural integrity of the data analysis and interpretation process.

Data Structures That Are Accountable to Indigenous Peoples and First Nations

This project was governed by a predominantly Indigenous research management group, with participation from all project investigators. The project was also guided by the strategic advice of three Indigenous 'critical friends' with national and international expertise in the fields of equity and higher education; Indigenous health and wellbeing; Indigenous education; and youth engagement. As such, there was a high degree of Indigenous representation within the project's data ecosystem, and the structures underpinning the use of project data, particularly through research analysis and knowledge translation processes. This way of working ensured that data structures were accountable to Indigenous peoples, and that data were protective and respective of their individual and collective interests.

Data That Is Protective and Respects Our Individual and Collective Interests

All Indigenous researchers in this project took part in making decisions about how data representing Indigenous people would be analysed and presented. It was agreed early in discussions that this project would be a qualitative study, whereby the views, perspectives and stories of Indigenous males attending, or who had completed university would be prioritised.

It was important to the research team that interviews were video-recorded, with a view to sharing vignettes from the interviews with other Indigenous stakeholders, particularly young Indigenous males contemplating higher education. Most participants embraced the opportunity to share their journey with others. Collecting stories in this way, with the intent of making them publicly available to a broader audience and to communicate these through university YouTube channels, was perceived as an effort to 'give back' to the community; it reflected a greater level of accountability to the participants; it made their voices more central to the project so that their words were not interpreted through the researchers; and simultaneously increased the potential to enhance community benefit. Unfortunately, due to COVID-19 there was insufficient time, and lack of funding to deliver on this aspect of the project. The team will continue to explore ways to use this data in a way that aligns with IDS, as opportunities arise.

Data That Is Contextual and Disaggregated (Available and Accessible at Individual, Community, and First Nations Levels)

An important part of choosing a qualitative design for this project was to provide a deeper level of context than what is typically captured through routine progress reporting completed by universities, and ultimately provided to the Australian Government as part of Indigenous and equity focused program funding arrangements. Previous research, which focused on the evaluation of Indigenous higher education programs, has been critical of quantitative data reporting as it has failed to contextualise the challenges faced by Indigenous higher education students (Smith et al., 2018), particularly concepts relating to academic success (Street et al., 2020). In particular, a greater appreciation of qualitative methodologies and evidence has been strongly advocated based on a study involving Indigenous scholars from all states and territories across Australia (Smith et al., 2018); other non-Indigenous scholars have also convincingly argued for the establishment of a decolonised data quality framework (Wilks et al., 2018).

A national workshop focused on articulating IDS principles in relation to Indigenous higher education has highlighted the importance of recognising sovereign rights, fostering Indigenous leadership, celebrating Indigenous expertise, and adopting a forward focus to improve Indigenous higher education outcomes (Smith et al., 2018). In our project, we aimed to address the abovementioned concerns from a strength-based perspective by privileging the voices of Indigenous males to provide first-hand contextual evidence about Indigenous male higher education.

In addition, it has also been acknowledged that gender is seldom considered in current routine reporting processes, which subsequently obscures the cumulative impacts of race and geographical remoteness from an intersectional lens. Our research helps to fill this void, with the planned development of vignettes honouring context, and including the voices of participants in a genuine and respectful way.

Data That Is Relevant and Empowers Sustainable Self-Determination and Effective Self-Governance

The fundamental premise of this project was to uncover, develop, and assist Indigenous males in sharing knowledge around which critical success factors and influences supported them to thrive and achieve in higher education. The idea was to draw on empirical research to identify strategies to help Indigenous males work effectively with fellow Indigenous males, families, community, Indigenous student services staff, and equity practitioners in higher education settings across Australia to increase rates of participation and completion among Indigenous males in higher education.

Hence, the project design and aims represent a move towards empowering sustainable self-determination, explicitly focusing on the voices of Indigenous males who are currently studying, or had recently completed, higher education. Indeed, the individual yarns were video recorded via Zoom with the intention of sharing these with a broader public audience. In that way, the identities of the participants were made public, and offered an opportunity to celebrate their achievements from a strengths-based perspective.

This model also ensured the relevance and sustainability of data long after completion of the research project, as the strategies can be used by relevant stakeholders to improve Indigenous male participation in higher education across Australia, and potentially in other countries with Indigenous populations.

Data Ownership

As per IDS principles, Indigenous peoples and communities should retain ownership of the data they provide to researchers; however, it is not always possible. For this project, Menzies School of Health Research legally retains the ownership of data. However, as Lovett et al. (2019) argue, a data governance mechanism was put in place to ensure that the data were used and held in a way that was acceptable to the participants and the broader community (Lovett et al., 2019). For this project, the intended data governance mechanism included publicly accessible vignettes of participants, to ensure that the project's legacy would benefit the community on an ongoing basis. As discussed above, this aspect of the project did not come to fruition. We also recognise that, despite good intentions, that this process was not equivalent to full IDS and ownership. However, within current legal limitations and the requirements of the funding body, we believed this to be the fullest extent to which we could give control over the data back to the concerned Indigenous stakeholders.

Implications for Policy and Practice

As discussed in a Chap. 8, education is a critical social determinant of health, particularly in the context of Indigenous health and wellbeing. While this chapter has focused on an education research project, the concepts of IDS could and should be applied to health promotion practice contexts as well. This could be achieved by directly engaging relevant Indigenous stakeholders in conceptualising, designing, collecting, analysis, and reporting of health data (Ray, 2016).

Engaging Indigenous stakeholders in the above-mentioned process will have two benefits (Griffiths & Smith, 2020; Ray, 2016). First, it will provide an opportunity for more meaningful information to be provided to relevant policymakers. Second, it will privilege the voices of Indigenous peoples to provide first-hand contextual evidence through research. This exercise will, in turn, provide opportunities for more open debates about the information needed to form the evidence base for Indigenous health promotion policy and practice, including that relating to young Indigenous males (Jansen, 2016; Ray, 2016). To address the intersections between health, equity, and education, access to and control of Indigenous health data by Indigenous peoples is essential (Gupta et al., 2021; Jansen, 2016). That is, addressing the nexus between health and education sectors is critical for promoting the optimal health and wellbeing of young men of colour (Gupta et al., 2021).

Conclusion

While scholarship on IDS has expanded rapidly over the past few years (Lovett et al., 2019), there are very few practical examples of how IDS principles can be applied purposefully in research, policy, and practice contexts, particularly in terms of research relating to young Indigenous males. In this chapter, we have explained how attempts were made to apply IDS principles during a qualitative research project relating to the experiences of Indigenous males pursuing, or who had completed, higher education.

We do not claim that this reflects a 'gold standard' or 'best practice.' Indeed, we faced many challenges. Rather, we intend to provide a practical example that can help guide others embarking on similar projects in health promotion and education research, policy, and practice spheres. The intention is to provoke debate and generate discussion regarding strengths-based approaches, to encourage reflection and continuous quality improvement across the education and health sectors, particularly as they relate to young Indigenous males. We encourage feedback of this nature.

Dedication

The research team would like to dedicate this chapter to a team member, Professor Dennis McDermott, who passed away over the course of the project. He was a strong supporter of strengthening Indigenous pathways to higher education, and his legacy lives on through the outcomes of this project.

References

Adams, M., Smith, J., & Fleay, J. (2021). How the practical perspectives of health impact on aboriginal males, family and communities. In B. Bennett (Ed.), *Aboriginal fields of practice*. Bloomsbury Publishing.

Australian Indigenous HealthInfoNet. (2018). *Overview of aboriginal and Torres Strait islander health status, 2017*. Australian Indigenous HealthInfoNet.

Australian Institute of Health and Welfare. (2012). *The health of Australia's men: A focus on five population groups. Cat. No. PHE160*. Australian Government.

Behrendt, L., Larkin, S., Griew, R., & Kelly, P. (2012). *Review of higher education access and outcomes for aboriginal and Torres Strait islander people: Final report*. Australian Government.

Bradley, D., Noonan, P., Nugent, H., & Scales, B. (2008). *Review of Australian higher education: Final report*. Commonwealth of Australia.

Department of Health. (2019). *National Men's health strategy 2020–2030. Commonwealth of Australia*. Australian Government.

Fogarty, W., Lovell, M., Langenberg, J., & Heron, M. J. (2018). *Deficit discourse and strengths-based approaches: Changing the narrative of aboriginal and Torres Strait islander health and wellbeing*. The Lowitja Institute.

Frawley, J., Smith, J., & Larkin, S. (2015). Beyond Bradley and Behrendt: Building a stronger evidence-base about indigenous pathways and transitions into higher education. *Learning Communities: International Journal of Learning in Social Contexts, 17*, 8–11.

Frawley, J., Ober, R., Olcay, M., & Smith, J. (2017). *Indigenous achievement in higher education and the role of self-efficacy: Rippling stories of success*. National Centre for Student Equity in Higher Education.

Frawley, J., Smith, J., & Larkin, S. (2017). Indigenous pathways, transitions and participation in higher education: From policy to practice. In J. Frawley, S. Larkin, & J. Smith (Eds.), *From policy to practice in higher education: Cross-cutting issues in indigenous pathways, transition and participation*. Singapore.

Griffiths, K., & Smith, J. (2020). Measuring health disparities in Australia: Using data to drive health promotion solutions. *Health Promotion Journal of Australia, 31*(2), 166–168. https://doi.org/10.1002/hpja.340

Gupta, H., Smith, J., Fleay, J., Lesiter, C. P. B., & Canuto, K. (2021). Understanding the nexus between alcohol consumption, social and emotional Well-being, and higher education outcomes among aboriginal and Torres Strait islander men in Australia. *International Journal of Mens Community and Social Health, 4*(1), e28–e37. https://doi.org/10.22374/ijmsch.v4i1.52

Jansen, R. (2016). Indigenous data sovereignty: A Māori health perspective. In T. Kukutai & J. Taylor (Eds.), *Indigenous data sovereignty: Toward an agenda* (pp. 192–211). ANU Press.

Lovett, R., Lee, V., Kukutai, T., Cormack, D., Rainie, S. C., & Walker, J. (2019). Good data practices for indigenous data sovereignty and governance. In A. Daly, S. K. Devitt, & M. Mann (Eds.), *Good Data* (pp. 26–36). Institute of Network Cultures.

Maiam Nayri Wingara. (2018, June 20). *Indigenous Data Sovereignty Communique.* Indigenous Data Sovereignty Summit held in Canberra.

Merlino, A., Smith, J., Adams, M., Bonson, J., Osborne, R., Judd, B., Drummond, M., Aanundsen, D., Fleay, J., & Christine, B. (2020). What do we know about the nexus between culture, age, gender and health literacy? Implications for improving the health and Well-being of young indigenous males. *International Journal of Men' Social and Community Health., 3*(2), e46–e57.

National Centre for Student Equity in Higher Education. (2018). *Building capacity and legacy workshop three: Indigenous perspectives of evaluation in higher education.* Curtin University.

Ray, L. (2016). Aboriginal and Torres Strait islander community wellbeing: Identified needs for statistical capacity. In T. Kukutai & J. Taylor (Eds.), *Indigenous data sovereignty: Toward an agenda* (pp. 213–231). ANU Press.

Shalley, F., Smith, J., Wood, D., Fredericks, B., & Robertson, K. (2019). *Understanding completion rates of indigenous higher education students from two regional universities: A cohort analysis.* National Centre for Student Equity in Higher Education.

Smith, J. (2018). A National Men's health strategy in Australia: Tips for implementation. *International Journal of Men's Social and Community Health, 1*(1), e15–e21.

Smith, J., Frawley, J., Pechenkina, E., Ludwig, W., Robertson, C., Gunstone, A., & Larkin, S. (2017). *Identifying strategies for promoting VET to higher education transitions for indigenous learners.* National Centre for Student Equity in Higher Education.

Smith, J., Adams, M., & Bonson, J. (2018). Investment in men's health in Australia. *Medical Journal of Australia, 208*(1), 6–7.

Smith, J., Pollard, K., Robertson, K., & Shalley, F. (2018). *Strengthening evaluation in indigenous higher education contexts in Australia: 2017 equity fellowship report.* National Centre for Student Equity in Higher Education.

Smith, J., Pollard, K., Robertson, K., & Trinidad, S. (2018). What do we know about evaluation in indigenous higher education contexts in Australia? *International Studies in Widening Participation, 4*(2), 18–31.

Smith, J., Drummond, M., Adams, M., Bonson, J., & Christie, B. (2019). Understanding inequities in men's health in Australia. In D. Griffith, M. Bruce, & R. Thorpe (Eds.), *Men's health equity: A handbook* (pp. 499–511). Routledge.

Smith, J. A., Gupta, H., Moore, S., Fleay, J., Stahl, G., Uink, B., Harvey, A., Radoll, P., Hill, B., Bennett, R., Vigona, J., & Merlino, A. (2022). Higher education aspirations, participation, and achievement of Australian indigenous males. Report prepared for the National Centre for Student Equity in Higher Education. Curtin University.

Smith, J., Merlino, A., Christie, B., Adams, M., Bonson, J., Osborne, R., Judd, B., Drummond, M., Aanundsen, D., & Fleay, J. (2020). "Dudes are meant to be tough as nails": The nexus between masculinities, culture, and health literacy from the perspective of young Aboriginal and Torres Strait Islander males – Implications for policy and practice. *American Journal of Men's Health. 14(3), 1–17.*

Stahl, G., McDonald, S., & Stokes, J. (2020). 'I see myself as undeveloped': Supporting indigenous first-in-family men in the transition to higher education. *Higher Education Research & Development, 39*(7), 1488–1501. https://doi.org/10.1080/07294360.2020.1728521

Street, C., Smith, J., Robertson, K., Guenther, J., Motlap, S., Ludwig, W., et al. (2020). Exploring definitions of success in Northern Territory indigenous higher education policy. *Journal of Educational Administration and History, 52*(4), 323–343. https://doi.org/10.1080/0022062 0.2020.1719391

The United Nations. (2007). 61/295. *United Nations Declaration of the Rights of Indigenous Peoples.*

Tomaszewski, W., Kubler, M., Perales, P., Western, M., Ramino, T., & Xiang, N. (2018). *Review of identified equity groups.* Institute for Social Science Research.

Walter, M., & Suina, M. (2019). Indigenous data, indigenous methodologies and indigenous data sovereignty. *International Journal of Social Research Methodology, 22*(3), 233–243.

Wilks, J., Kennedy, G., Drew, N., & Wilson, K. (2018). Indigenous data sovereignty in higher education: Towards a decolonised data quality framework. In I. Dobson (Ed.), *Australian universities' review.* Melbourne.

Wood, D., Fredericks, B., Smith, J., Watkin-Lui, F., Larkin, S., Gruppetta, M., … Rigney, L.-I. (2019). *Addressing the gap between policy and implementation: strategies for improving the educational outcomes of Indigenous students. Final report prepared for the Office of Learning and Teaching.*

Chapter 10
La Cultura Cura and *El Joven Noble*: Culturally Rooted Theory and Practice Formulations for Healing Wounded Boys and Young Men of Colour in the United States

Heriberto Escamilla, R. Bong Vergara, Jerry Tello, and Héctor Sánchez-Flores

Cada cabeza es un mundo: An Introduction

On the surface, this chapter is about healing the self-destructive behaviour of Indigenous and Latinx Boys and Young Men of Colour (BYMOC) in the U.S. and guiding them toward lives that honour both their ancestors and descendants. Implicitly, it is also an exploration of the limitations of the written word – how effectively meaning can be faithfully articulated and respectfully conveyed across different realities. From 2006 to 2019, we were blessed to host, assist, and translate for a *Wirrarika* elder and medicine man called *Ri'tak'ameh*[1] as he helped heal hundreds of people throughout California, Arizona, and Nevada. We observed that most of the people he treated changed in some positive way, even if they did not completely understand the inner workings of his treatment. After his interventions, their faces were less tense than before and their physical movements were lighter. Wary of our own bias, we confirmed observations with subjects and other witnesses. In doing so, we realised that our capacity to understand and explain the healing

---

[1] *Ri'taka'meh*, a medicine man, was from a small community in the Sierra Madre Occidental. His "traditions" were handed down to him for his people. He shared them with us *te'wari* (outsiders) reluctantly and fully aware of his transgression. We are forever indebted to him and his family. Out of respect for him and his people, we share his Indigenous name only.

H. Escamilla · R. B. Vergara · J. Tello (✉) · H. Sánchez-Flores
National Compadres Network, San Jose, CA, USA
e-mail: heriberto.escamilla@compadresnetwork.org; tellojt@compadresnetwork.org;
hsf@compadresnetwork.org

"mechanism" were challenged by our facility with language. We were also challenged by the boundaries established by the respective cultures in which we were raised. We lived in different realities – not perspectives, nor theories – but realities.

In this chapter, we speak for Latinx, Mexican American, Chicano, and Indigenous BYMOC in the United States, and while our instinct is to include the familiar, realities are different. The human impact of genocide of people from the land that was previously Mexico, which is now the United States, is not the same as that for the enslavement of Africans. The experience of Mexicans after the Mexican-American War differs from that of more recent immigrants from Guatemala, Honduras, El Salvador, and other Central American countries. The experience of our relatives from other corners of the earth are also distinct. Science complicates our task by insisting that true understanding comes primarily, and some would even say exclusively, through dissecting and analysing – through specificity.

We claim a *mechicano indio*[2] philosophical and cultural foundation in speaking to the interconnectedness that unites us. The Indigenous people of Meso-America developed and used two calendar systems for making sense of the world. On the one hand, the 365-day *Xiuhpohualli* monitored the sun, seasons and was consulted on physical matters, like agriculture; on the other hand, the 260-day *Tonalpohualli* monitored the manifestations of the soul and was consulted on spiritual concerns that influenced thinking, feeling, and behaviour. We take this two-calendar system as a reminder of the duality[3] of life and health – that illness and wellness are simultaneously and inseparably physical and spiritual. As noted, bridging the many realities that constitute life through words is a daunting task. But we take heart in the words that our brother, *Ri'ta'kame*, left with us – *le hacemos la lucha:* we'll put up a battle for the young people whose spirits we call back to the circle.

El Hombre Propone, Dios Dispone: The Proposal

We propose that the self-destructive behaviour of many BYMOC is a misguided attempt to heal woundedness. We subscribe to the term intergenerational trauma to convey the current understanding that, for people of colour, woundedness could be more appropriately seen as violent, terrorizing, and painful disconnections that have

---

[2] People often associate the Méxica or Aztecs as representative of Meso-American culture and thought. While their contributions were undoubtedly important, many philosophical concepts have been traced back to and perhaps beyond the Olmeca, often considered the Mother Culture of Mexico. Many of the concepts we utilize are common from the Ra'ramuri and Yaqui of the north, Wirrarika and as far down as the Quiche people of the Yucatan.

[3] Duality is perhaps the most common theme in Indigenous, Meso-American philosophy. Examples of this are found in the *Popul Vu*, sacred book of the Maya narrates the exploits of the sacred twins as they recover the bones of their ancestors. Among the Tolteca, Quetzalcoatl was at once an actual person and title conferred to one that had integrated earth and sky, represented by a plumed serpent with a head at both ends. The main deity in the Nahua pantheon was *Ometeotl*, which translates very roughly as Two God.

occurred over the last 500 years and exacerbated by present-day inequalities and stressors. Given the racially motivated violence that has stewed for centuries and erupted most recently in 2020, we believe the time is ripe for serious consideration of different solutions.

While impossible to establish exact numbers, recent estimates claim that as many as 56 million lives were lost in the century following the European arrival in the Americas (Koch et al., 2019). Historians tell us the violence manifested in many forms – from homicide, uprooting children from family and community, forced labour, and enslavement to the destruction of sacred places of worship – sparking cataclysmic loss and suffering by native peoples. While in current Western clinical terms, the resultant condition among survivors could be understood as Post Traumatic Stress Disorder (PTSD) (Williams et al., 2017), we prefer the term 'woundedness' because it more accurately conveys the pain and collective *susto*[4] – the terror that overwhelmed individuals, families, and communities over generations. Similarly, Brave Heart et al. (2011) uses the term 'soul wounds' to emphasize that the damage affects all aspects of the person—from thinking to feeling, behaviour, and spirit.

Another critical point is that soul woundedness is transmitted to successive generations. We are convinced that one mechanism for its transmission is our disconnection from all that makes us whole, including the natural environment that nurtures us. Wounded parents—those who are isolated, depressed, drug-abusing, frustrated, overworked, traumatized, etc. – also wound their children. They hurt children with the words and feelings they project, the values they teach, and their day-to-day interactions. Seemingly oblivious to that reality, current interventions of youth-serving institutions rarely include parents and families. In fact, in a recent listening tour of seven U.S. communities, youth tell us they feel neither represented nor supported, but rather punished by the institutions that have been established to serve them.

When the youth are abused and traumatized at home and in their communities, should it be a surprise that they are overwhelmed with pain and ill-equipped to cope adaptively? They become trapped in a loop of high-risk behaviours. The numbers are clear: Blacks, Latinos, Indigenous and BYMOC, in general, are grossly over-represented in correctional institutions (Dragomir & Tadros, 2020; Jeffers, 2019; Kovera, 2019), bear a disproportionate share of school suspensions, are exposed to excessively violent interactions with police, and surrounded by cultural cues that diminish their identity, damage their self-worth, and condition self-destruction.

In this chapter, we focus our attention on boys and youths of colour, with the understanding that both illness and wellbeing are best understood as *relational*. As

---

[4] *Susto* literally translates as "fright" into English. It is often dismissed as a culture-bound condition, specific to Mexico and other Central American countries. While it is often dismissed, a careful study of the physical symptomology reveals that it is a different culturally rooted understanding of a condition very similar to PTSD. The condition is similar to other Indigenous formulations around the world. We recognize it as a valid and legitimate condition that has been devalued by researchers and practitioners with cursory understandings of its origins and associated practices.

an individual heals, so too does the circle, community and society in which they live. Nonetheless, research indicates that young boys of colour are exposed to higher rates of trauma than other demographics groups (Graham et al., 2017). Moreover, youth of colour are both perpetrators and victims of violence at disproportionally higher rates than other demographic groups (CDC, 2003). Whether we choose to understand the transmission of woundedness as modelling, behaviour reinforcement, or other culturally accepted constructs, boys and youth of colour are trapped in a world of pain, fear and violence. With this in mind, we propose a culturally-rooted way of understanding trauma, its long-term consequences and an intervention that helps young men, feel wanted, transform their pain into compassion, reconnect with their authentic self, and join the circle of life.

Current Practice Concerns in Latinx, Mexican American, and Chicano Communities

Research supports the idea that woundedness, more clinically known as a disorder, anxiety, or depression, may indeed be an antecedent of self-destructive behaviour. Substance dependence, depression, acute stress disorder, disruptive behaviour disorders in children (e.g., conduct disorder and oppositional defiance), phobias, sleep disorders (Coll et al., 2012) and post-traumatic stress disorder (PTSD) are thought to be associated with criminal behaviour (Gibson et al., 1999; Maschi et al., 2008; Spitzer et al., 2001; Wolff & Shi, 2010) and have been suggested to intensify high-risk behaviour, including status offenses (e.g., substance abuse, persistent disobedience, curfew violations, and habitual truancy) (Vanden WallBake, 2013) and illegal offenses (e.g., crimes against a person, inchoate crimes, statutory crimes, crimes against property) (Ardino, 2012).

Research also suggests that Latinx, Mexican Americans, and Chicanos are especially vulnerable to these soul wounds and their transmission across generations because of multiple stressors, including political violence in their home countries and trauma during migration (Cerdeña et al., 2021), settlement-related stress (Santiago et al., 2018), and parenting stress that leads to competence problems for children (Cabrera & Hennigar, 2019). Researchers are also showing a growing interest in intergenerational trauma as a means of understanding stress and wellbeing in Latinx populations (Cerdeña et al., 2021; Isobel et al., 2019). However, much remains unclear about its dynamics, and a better understanding might inform strategies and interventions for resolving the impacts of trauma in Latinx, Mexican American, and Chicano communities (Cerdeña et al., 2021; Orozco-Figueroa, 2021). The escalation of violent, trauma-inducing, anti-Latino and anti-immigrant racism in the U.S. and the increasing frequency of damaging contact with immigration authorities, police, and justice systems make it imperative to develop robust frameworks for understanding.

Addressing the omission of macro-level risk factors for intergenerational trauma is a vital point for discussion. Most current research literature on intergenerational trauma in Latinx, Mexican American, and Chicano communities focuses on individual risk factors at the expense of structural, social, and cultural forces that also shape behaviour (Cerdeña et al., 2021). For example, research on Mexican American and Chicano adolescents shows that promoting family values, strong ethnic identity, and the use of cultural strengths supports adaptive coping, reduces adolescent problem behaviours (Gonzales et al., 2012) and mitigates the cycle of intergenerational trauma. Gonzales et al. (2020) found that the Coping Orientation to Problems Experienced (COPE) Inventory was not a good fit, while collectivist coping strategies resonated better with Latinx youth, suggesting that relationship- and culture-based approaches to coping could be more appropriate. Furthermore, Andrade et al. (2020) found that deeper ethnic pride and belonging weakened the impact of perceived racial/ethnic discrimination on mental health, suggesting that culturally rooted interventions are more effective for Latinx, Mexican Americans, and Chicanos.

Given the macro-level dimensions of intergenerational trauma, the practice field needs a comprehensive understanding of cultural root-causes of intergenerational trauma for programs to effectively bring not only health but also hope to vulnerable Latinx, Mexican American, and Chicano communities. We contend that BYMOC need youth development practices that are culturally rooted and meaningful to them. We discuss below the conceptual framework for such a practice for Latinx, Mexican American, and Chicano communities.

La Cultura Cura: Culture as Medicine

Cultura or culture generally refers to the customs and behaviours of people unified through history, language and geography. Our understanding is similar to that expressed by Kluckhohn and Strodtbeck (1961), who saw culture as a set of solutions to basic existential problems. In small groups, values are passed down through personal interactions, with bigger societies preserving and transmitting it through institutions (Hofstede & Hofstede, 2010). Our working definition of *cultura* refers to a dynamic set of orienting *valores* (values), passed down from one generation to the next, which are a source of cultural identity, and serve as mechanisms for maintaining interconnectedness, individual health, and family wellbeing. Culture also includes our relationship to that which we may not understand but is nonetheless vital – the spiritual domain of life. In the Americas, our Indigenous ancestors acknowledged, respected, and revered the sacredness of their relationship to all forms of life, including the physical forces that support existence – earth, wind, water, and fire. This appreciation of the interconnectedness of life is one of the main characteristics of what we respectfully call an Indigenous reality. Tello (2018) uses the term *Tloque Nahuaque*[5] to convey that sense of sacred interconnectedness, the organizing idea in our philosophy.

La Cultura Cura (LCC) is an Indigenous knowledge-based framework for understanding the cultural grounding of health and for addressing self-destructive behaviour and its associated thinking and feeling processes. In the literature, LCC can be traced back to what researchers call *indigenismo,* a Civil Rights Era attempt to acknowledge, reclaim, and reconnect people of Mexican and Central American descent to their Indigenous roots devastated by colonisation (Orozco-Figueroa, 2021). The formal foundation of LCC began with a 1988 gathering of nineteen Chicano, Native, Latino community advocates and social service providers. Led by Jerry Tello, Ricardo Carrillo, Jésus de la Rosa, Isaac Cardenas and others, the group developed the basic tenets of LCC to serve others by committing to first addressing their own colonised pain and self-destructive behaviour. The culturally rooted, inside-out understanding of healing as reconnection with authentic self, family, and community was our alternative to the dominant approach, which we believe sees healing mostly as alleviating physical and observable symptoms – an approach analogous to turning off a smoke alarm to extinguish a fire. Applied originally to high-risk Latinx, Mexican American, and Chicano male youth, LCC has since been extended as an effective tool for youth of colour, in general.

Four Valores

LCC defines four core *valores* (values) underlying behaviour, dignity, respect, love, and trust (Table 10.1). Each value has a central proposition that is effectuated by a target process, which in turn, results in a target outcome. The overarching goal is to re-root the adolescent in these core values so they may serve as medicine.[6] Jerry Tello articulates the organizing principle of LCC as, "Within the collective Dignity, Respect, Love and Trust of all people exists as the pathway to beautiful harmonious life." It reflects the idea that all people carry within themselves the medicine necessary to heal from the overwhelming effects of trauma and other forms of violence.

LCC asserts that medicine is embedded in Indigenous culture, in Indigenous knowledge systems, wisdom, music, dance, and especially ritual and ceremony.

---

[5] Sometimes seen as *En Tloque Nahuaque*, *Tloque Nahuaque* is from Nahuatl, one of the major Indigenous languages spoken by the people of Central Mexico. There is considerable debate as to the precise meaning of the term. Suggested possibilities include "the lord of the near and the nigh," that which is far and that which is close or to one side. Others argue it is a name that refers to Mexica deities such as Ometeotl or Tezcatlipoca or an epithet that conveys the omnipresence of the ultimate deity.

[6] The term medicine is commonly used in Native American and other Indigenous conceptions of health. According to Merriam-Webster, the term has Latin origins and therefore calls for some discussion. According to most sources, medicine refers to treatment with great care and skill. It refers to the treatment and not so much a substance, as commonly understood in conventional language.

Table 10.1   The four core *La Cultura Cura valores* (values) and their central propositions, target processes, and target outcomes

Valor/Value	Proposition	Target process	Target outcome
Dignidad (dignity)	The youth should feel like the sacred blessings that they are.	Adolescent is made to genuinely feel welcomed for who they are.	The deep sense of connectedness and community cultivates.
Respeto (respect)	Everyone has a sacred purpose in life, defined as an inherent sense of value that is secured even before one finds his/her place and value in a social sense.	A sense of responsibility for one's ethnic community, family, and personal self-worth is built in a group setting, driving growth and self-betterment through culturally rooted mentorship.	Adolescent builds meaning in service of self, family, and ethnic community. Finding, claiming, and fulfilling one's sacred purpose results in *respeto*.
Cariño (love)	Everyone has indigenous ancestral values, teachings, and medicine that can guide, support, and heal themselves and their communities.	Self-healing is mediated by ritual and traditional ceremonies, leading to an internalization of ancestral values, beliefs, and indigenous teachings, thus, a positive love and vision of heritage and community.	The adolescent's internalization of indigenous ancestral values, beliefs, and indigenous teachings guide, support, and facilitate healing of self and others in a compassionate and culturally rooted way.
Confianza (trust)	Everyone should have a safe, trusted place, and people where and to whom they could turn for growth, support. We heal ourselves as we heal our peers, family members, and the larger community.	Through culturally rooted mentorship and ongoing engagement in community activities, embolden spirit of the adolescent so he/she can overcome life's pressures with sure-footedness.	Access to a safe, trusted place, and people for growth, support, and healing raises hope, enabling the adolescent to approach life with confidence. Emergent self-betterment is acknowledged so it takes root.

LCC also asserts that healing is reciprocal: just as people can cause harm to one another, so, too, can an individual's self-healing facilitate the healing of the people with whom they are in relationship. Unlike Western medicine that views healing as the application of clinical therapies, LCC views healing as a shared cultural experience – it is relational, occurring in our communion with others.

The Medicine Wheel: Mapping the Healing Journey

LCC defines both a structure and a process for healing. The healing process has five stages in which fear and pain are transformed into increased appreciation for the subjective experience of self and others (see Fig. 10.1). The stage model is similar

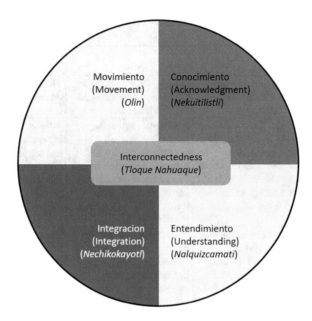

Fig. 10.1 La Cultura Cura's medicine wheel

to and includes all of the elements proposed by Prochaska and Velicer (1997) but acknowledges the subjective fear that keeps people from moving, and includes a cultural/spiritual element to which BYMOC more readily respond.

Moreover, the process is cyclical, suggesting that wounds heal slowly and are difficult to eliminate definitively, and that we revisit wounds to understand them from a more adaptive perspective. Indeed, it is by staying in contact with wounded-ness that people develop compassion and understanding of others. LCC's version of the medicine wheel[7] helps us understand the process by which the interaction of acknowledgment, understanding, integration, movement, and interconnectedness contribute to healing. This medicine wheel underlies the LCC curricula, strategies, and interventions.

Conocimiento (Acknowledgment)

Many Latinx, Mexican American, and Chicano youth come from families who have experienced generations of racism, discrimination, and oppression. In response, they detach from their connection to themselves, their families, their relationships, and their own behaviours. They may conform to cultural stereotypes of masculinity

---

[7] While the colours, associated animals, symbols and even direction of movement may vary, the medicine wheel is common to virtually all Indigenous peoples of the Americas. Formed by the path of the sun across the surface of the earth, it can serve as an orienting tool that guides our movement through life.

and femininity or internalize negative images of themselves. The safety and security of the *círculo* helps them face and overcome tendencies to run, fight or push people away. The consistent and dependable structure of the *círculo* becomes the container that allows people to feel welcomed, accepted and wanted.

Entendimiento (Understanding)

Once youth are grounded, they begin to resonate with the teachings offered in the *circulo*. The facilitator, peers and lessons touch their hearts. Youth that are accustomed to survival mode experience the opportunity for reflection, assessment and understanding. They become emotionally engaged, allowing them to discover, rediscover or reaffirm values they carry within themselves. They also learn to appreciate the importance of ceremonial life and understand its use in maintaining well-being. In this stage, they also begin giving voice to the *cargas* (emotional baggage) they carry and to tolerate the discomfort and pain of changing self-destructive thinking and action. In doing so, they begin bonding with others and experience *confianza* (trust).

Integracion (Integration)

Applying the principle of *en lak'ech,*[8] youth learn to pay close attention to the effects of their actions on others. They develop *palabra* (credible word), being careful that their words are not used to hurt others, being honest with their skills and capacities so that they live up to what they say and do not over-promise or deceive. In this stage of the process, young people start integrating recently discovered *regalos* (gifts, e.g., skills and abilities), providing a foundation for lives that are self-fulfilling and of service to others. This ability to put things together, to synthesize is the basis of respect and dignity and discovering their sacred purpose.[9]

Movimiento (Movement)

In this stage, young people begin to "move." They exhibit new behaviours that expose them to their own self-judgment as well as criticism from others. At this stage, youth need support in committing to their new ways of being and expressing themselves. Learning to commit, to have palabra and work when times get tough is

---

[8] *En lak'ech* is a greeting from the Mayan Language that has gained widespread popularity of late. Literally, it translates as "you are my other me." LCC uses the term to promote interconnectedness, respect and affection between people.

[9] A thorough discussion of the term "sacred" would take volumes and well beyond our scope. We respectfully offer the following definition: "*Sacred* refers to that which us set apart, cannot be completely understood nor explained and related with the ultimate source of life."

a critical step in healing. They need the participation of family and relationships that witness and continue to support the transition. They experience interconnectedness and *ganas*,[10] which allows them make sense of their lives.

En Tloque Nahuaque (Interconnected Sacredness)

The final step of the healing process, like all significant accomplishments in life, is an ongoing process and never a destination. When our brother *Ri'taka'me* embarked on a trip with us, his refrain was always the same, *"a ver hasta donde llegamos"* ("let's see how far we get"). Having given voice or expressed the pain of disconnection, re-rooted in the values embedded in culture and transmitted through relationships, youth are better equipped to battle the challenges of daily life and their transition to manhood. In this stage, it is critical that youth continue to strengthen their commitment to healing themselves and their relations. As evidence of our commitment, we invite graduates to be part of our extended kinship network.

La Cultura Cura's Practice Intervention: *El Joven Noble*

With *La Cultura Cura* as the underlying philosophical premise, *El Joven Noble* is a youth-development, support, and character development program for BYMOC aged 10–24 years. *El Joven Noble* consists of a 12-week curriculum focused on healing the results of intergenerational trauma and re-rooting young men in their Indigenous values. The program is relationship-based, reconnecting BYMOC to their true potential as *jovenes nobles,* or noble youth (Fig. 10.2).

Table 10.2 distils NCN's experience with Latinx, Mexican American, and Chicano youth into a program framework, which shows that with cultural disconnection comes an eroded (a) sacred purpose, (b) sense of responsibility, (c) interdependence, (d) development, and (e) enthusiasm. This erosion is mitigated and ultimately reversed by the practical use of *mechicano indio* rituals, rite of passage ceremonies, and traditional practices. The feedback loop accounts for the cycle of learning and re-learning when addressing issues of development, adverse behaviour and negative thoughts, feelings, and perceptions among Latinx, Mexican American, and Chicano youth. It does so by putting to practical therapeutic use the nurturing capacity of community elders and family members.

El Joven Noble makes practical use of five teachings in facilitating rites of passage from childhood to manhood, positing that their erosion aggravates personal, family, and community dysfunction. Table 10.2 outlines the five teachings that guide a noble youth—sacred purpose, sense of responsibility, interdependence, development, and enthusiasm. Each teaching has a proposition that is effectuated by a target process and results in a target outcome.

---

[10] *Ganas* is a common term used in Mexican Spanish. It refers to both the willingness and energy to move – to accomplish something.

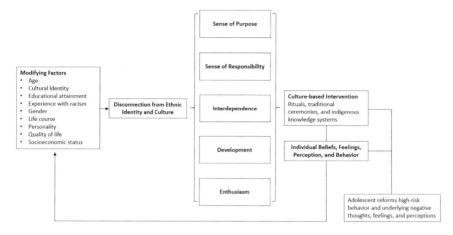

Fig. 10.2   El Joven Noble Program Framework for Culturally Rooted Healing

Table 10.2   The five core foci of *El Joven Noble* and their central propositions, target processes, and target outcomes

Teachings	Proposition	Target Process	Target Outcome
Sacred purpose	A sense of accomplishment from expressed service and articulated purpose are rooted in ethnic identity.	Group recognizes adolescent's accomplishment, which sustains transformational self-healing.	Adolescent builds meaning in service of self, family, and ethnic community.
Responsibility	Self-betterment is a healthy, adaptive, and culturally rooted response to the need to overcome life's struggles.	A sense of responsibility for one's ethnic community is built, driving growth and self-betterment.	Adolescent gains control over own functioning in a way that reflects ethnic identity.
Interdependence	Adolescent needs to develop trust and interdependence with peers, family members, and the larger community in order to grow.	Growth leads to re-integration with the positive vision of the community, which in turn leads to interdependence.	The cycle of violence is disrupted by an interdependence with the community.
Development	Guiding young men of colour follows a circular process of sharing, learning, and re-learning.	Adolescent and elders commune with *cariño* (love) to offer indigenous knowledge that focus healing.	Adolescent builds ethnic pride, develops respect for others, and learns to cope with intergroup differences.
Enthusiasm	The raising of hope allows an individual to approach life with *ganas* (enthusiasm).	Through ongoing community events, embolden spirit of the adolescent so s/he can overcome life's pressures.	Emergent leadership capacity and self-betterment by the adolescent are acknowledged so they take root.

El Joven Noble and Círculo

Tello and NCN staff adapted the universal practice of sitting in circle (*circulo*) to eat, talk, celebrate, and mourn life as a tool for healing young men, women, and families. Each círculo session revolves around a specific Indigenous knowledge-based teaching. The teaching refers to one or more specific values, such as respect, accountability, and palabra (credible word). In addition, the teaching may have an associated *manualidad*[11] or craft that engages and reinforces the teaching. In each session, participants are provided the opportunity to check-in and acknowledge their current reality, as well as the challenges and accomplishments they are facing. In Indigenous ways, this process of sitting, being present and listening to others, is a way of honouring them. Through speaking aloud, participants share and release physical/spiritual baggage, and connect with others. Experience and research tell us that active, non-judging listening is an important skill in the development of empathy among youth (Jones et al., 2019). This is used in all círculo sessions, whether to check-in or to reflect on teachings. Each *círculo* series ends with a formal celebration, attended by participant relatives and significant others that witness, validate and help reinforce the participant's commitments.

Facilitators and Training

While the culturally rooted curriculum provides a context and engages youth, the role of facilitators as supportive and caring guides cannot be underestimated. The training is open to all, but usually attracts people in the "helping professions," such as counsellors, therapists, educators, probation officers. Joven Noble was originally designed for young men, and we've found that young men from similar backgrounds as participants are the best "fit," but gender is not a deterrent. What's more important is that facilitators commit to "walking the talk" – to living the values they teach. Potential facilitators undergo a highly interactive and rigorous three-day training, conducted in círculo format. A ten-item "healing-informed skills" scale in development is used to assess the facilitators' comfort with questions such as listening without explaining, sharing from their own experience, dealing with participants that digress from the process, dealing with the spiritual aspects of the círculo, feeling emotional during sessions, or creating a space where people feel encouraged to share.

Trained facilitators are invited and encouraged to join the NCN kinship network, where they can continue learning from others, and share their gifts and find support when needed, and they are encouraged to maintain contact for technical assistance. In an informal follow-up study of 130 people trained in all NCN curricula during the

---

[11] *Manualidad* is a common term for a handicraft. The hand in Meso-American culture is the instrument through which we express the intentions of our heart. *Manualidades* result in hand made concrete outcomes, something participants can take pride in making.

last 6 months of 2019 immediately prior to the COVID-19 pandemic, we found that facilitators ranged in age from 23 to 69, with an average age of 43. They represented 113 zip codes across nine (9) American states.

Figure 10.3 abstracts this dialogue-based, culturally rooted therapeutic process in a Theory of Change. It is defined by the idea that young men need other men, their family, and community to prepare for manhood. As a rites of passage program, *El Joven Noble* takes account the quality of an adolescent's bond with his relations, the strength of his ethnic identity, and his self-efficacy in applying positive Indigenous-based masculinity ideals to his transition from childhood to manhood– (1) palabra (credible word), (2) not bringing harm to others, (3) taking responsibility for self and others in his circle, and (4) making time to reflect, prayer and ceremony (5) being a positive example. Figure 10.4 illustrates how the two interventions in Fig. 10.3 lead to the expected outcomes.

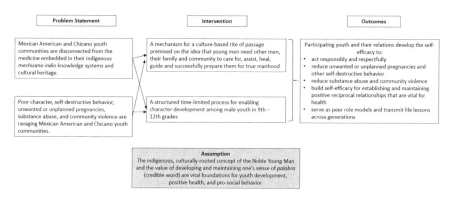

Fig. 10.3 El Joven noble theory of change

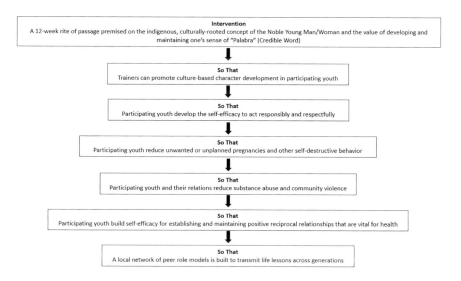

Fig. 10.4 El Joven noble outcome chain

Evidence of Program Efficacy

NCN has been conducting in person círculos, training facilitators, building capacity and providing technical assistance since 1988. In addition to our internal evaluation, much of the work has been assessed and highlighted in other reports such as those cited below. We should also note that beginning in March 2020, NCN like many organizations adapted their work to meet COVID-19 restrictions. This was especially significant for us because our indigenous-based practices promoted the importance of physical space, respect for the elements, face-to-face contact and interaction. Maintaining the spirit of our work in a virtual format was challenging, but we did our best, *le hicimos la lucha*. Many of collaborators, especially Native peoples patiently wait for a return to "normal."

Some participants, especially those that experienced the face-to-face format, noted the difference between those and virtual círculos. A few others have noted that the virtual format actually helps those people that would be reluctant to share in person. At best, we have very preliminary feedback in both directions and not enough experience with both formats to offer a more informed assessment the effectiveness of virtual círculos.

Recent projects include a five-year collaboration with Race Forward that was funded by the California Endowment. NCN provided in-person training and technical assistance to 140 institutional policy makers and practitioners in Salinas, California in response to a rash of violence and police shootings of several people of colour. The interventions were part of a larger effort for making meaningful change between residents and the institutions that serve them. A project report by Bradshaw-Dieng et al. (2016) found this quote by the mayor of Salinas City poignant to add: "[the city manager] referred to [NCN's work] as diversity, and I said no, this is different. This is a new framework. We are making a shift." As part of that shift, Motivating Individual Leadership for Public Advancement (MILPA) and Building Health Communities (BHC) led a campaign under this framework to get the Monterey County board of supervisors to unanimously approve reducing the beds in a newly planned juvenile hall from 150 to 120.

In addition to wide acceptance by community-based organizations and juvenile justice departments, NCN has worked with public and private school systems nationally in southern California, northern California, Maryland, and Texas, to operationalize LCC into the education field. Several of these partners have become anchor organizations that have either institutionalized *El Joven Noble* or continued to train facilitators on a regular basis.

In 2017, NCN provided training and technical assistance on *El Joven Noble*, Circle Keeping for educators in the Coachella Unified School District in southern California. Between 2018 and 2019, *El Joven Noble* prepared youth to conduct a Youth Participatory Action Project (YPAR) in three communities: San Jose and San Diego in California, and Denver, Colorado.

Between December 2017 and January 2018, NCN provided training for 64 service providers as part of a larger projected implemented by the Gang Reduction

Office of Los Angeles, California. The services included *El Joven Noble* sessions for 64 attendees and follow-up Circle Keeper training for 31 of those participants. Program evaluation of the in-person work reflected positive feedback, prompting the project manager to note:

> I think that when it comes to NCN, a lot of the agency personnel really liked their training a lot. It resonated with them in many ways. Not to the point where people felt equipped to start their own circles, but it was something that they did find useful, so I think we did start the process of our service providers starting their own healing, so a few of them will go to their own circle on their own time, and that's a step in the right direction.

Empirical Evidence of Program Efficacy

To date, NCN has conducted Circle Keeper/facilitator trainings in over 40 cities. Follow-up with facilitators trained in 2019, immediately before the COVID-19 pandemic, indicated that 74% went on to implement at least one círculo for a total of 5460 participants. While we assist and consult with projects that implement NCN, we rely heavily on external evaluations, as alluded to above. In addition to this validation, we also assess our success using what people tell us in their own words. While tedious and time consuming, these methods are more consistent with our culture-based approach. The data presented below were collected from a sample of eight students that participated in a virtual version of *El Joven Noble* between 2018 and 2019 at a San Jose high school. All respondents identified as male, ranging from 18 to 22 years in age.

Círculo Experience

A few respondents noted that the círculo helped them manage pandemic-related stress from isolation. One noted that the virtual experience was not the same as the in-person experience. He noted that for him, the "intimacy" was not the same, but the "idea and concept" was nonetheless present and overall helpful. The same responded also liked the "virtual" format, indicating that it allows people to "show their true selves." The virtual format helps participants feel less "judged," less "shy" and open to talking. Another participant differentiated between his experience with the círculo and on-line school sessions. He found the círculo much more enjoyable than school.

Acceptance; You are a Blessing

One young man described the círculo as "open arms," and "welcomed by people that I didn't even know." Another participant noted the círculo was:

[A]bout trust and honouring people that are there for you. I never really had that. I didn't trust nobody and didn't want to talk to nobody. But when I started going to the circle that's the main thing that I took away from there, was to start trusting people and to start having respect for the people that love me.

Another respondent offered that the círculo helped him manage the stress that he attributed to the isolation and the pandemic. Another learned the importance of "being honest" and "respectful to others."

Confianza/Trust

A common theme that emerged from the interviews was *confianza*/trust in who they were, perhaps less willing to follow along with others, but to lead. One respondent noted that he learned quite a bit about public speaking, suggesting a greater sense of competency and confidence. He expressed gratitude to the círculo facilitators. Another young man told us that the círculo helped him:

[S]ee things as more valuable, like trust and respect, because trust is needed now between one person to another because of what's happening with the virus. People need to trust one another and tell people who they are, they need to respect the person's boundaries, the limits, also responsibility of who you are. I would say I am better overall. I am not as mischievous as I use to be, and I don't look for trouble like I use to. I know that there [are] better things out there. With my friends I kind of overlooked them, I stepped away from them, I kinda knew how they were, I follow my own thing now. I am not so much a follower now; more so a leader now.

Relationships and Respect

The importance of relationship, while not always mentioned directly by the young men is evident throughout the responses. One participant noted that he was impressed with how the maestros, (teacher) or in this case círculo facilitators treated participants with respect. This modelling helped him adopt a "more respectful attitude toward others." One young man detailed how his relationship with facilitators and group experience helped him change his relationship with his mother:

Yeah, with my mom, me and her didn't have a good connection, she disowned me when I was 13, and I really didn't have no respect for her. But when I started going to the circle and started talking to Ariel, Mickey, and people that ran the circle, I actually opened up to them and it just taught me to look at her shoes and I went over to my moms and told her I was sorry, and she said sorry. Now we have a good connection and more than it was. I relate to my parents. I respect them, I treat them like I want to be treated, in a good way. My uncle, he's going through a class, he's changed a lot, and I changed a lot during this class and he's changing more during the period he's taken the class. I really relate to him.

Interconnection

Relatedly, another participant was particularly impacted by the concept of *en lak'ech*. Translated from the Mayan as "you are my other me," this common greeting between people emphasizes the importance of acceptance, compassion and empathy. For example. One young man noted the importance of words – what one says. The lesson he learned was that "what I say actually hurts people and that sometimes people work hard for some things that other people don't have, and [that] makes them feel that they are guilty of something I have not done yet, and makes me want to learn more about it."

One of the young men responded on romantic relationships, noting that:

> [I]t doesn't matter who you get, if you get someone, you should love them for who they are, not for what you want them to be. Yes definitely, it brought me insight to my own personal values especially with family and friends, like being kind and understanding of others, and like for example one of the biggest one is maintaining and keeping healthy relationships. With not just boyfriends and girlfriends, but with family and friends and co-workers. I felt the whole group was moving on even if a person joined the call late or missed it, the next call we would make him feel like he was in that (missed) class. That's what's good about the class, we didn't leave anybody behind, if someone missed the class, we made them feel like they were actually in the class, which felt great.

Changing Values and Enduring Change

In addition to changing behaviours and attitudes, respondents were asked if their participation resulted in changes in their personal values. Their responses strongly suggest that the participant's experience in the círculo, especially their interactions with facilitators and peers generalized to values with respect to family, school and peers. One participant made this connection in this way:

> Family is important. It definitely got stronger through círculo. The way I think of them is that they are one big family, you can always come to them for anything you need or anyone you want to talk to. They are always there for you. That is the same like my family and your family, you always have their support and that is why I look at it like that.

A second young man highlighted a profound change in what he considered important:

> They really changed things a lot. It made me rethink my whole system, reset the way I do things. I value more what my parents have done, what my family is going through. I really appreciate what they are doing to get me to a better future. Before this class I would be a person who would make hate speech and comments, but now, during the class I see ways in a different way, and a different point of view. I see a lot of things I shouldn't have said, a lot of things I regret. When I would be with my friends before the virus came in, I would be a disrespectful person, untrustworthy. Now I feel more better, a trustworthy person, a person of confianza.

Discussion

The theoretical and practice formulations behind LCC and *El Joven Noble* have implications for practice, policy, and research in health and youth development disciplines. In clinical practice, they demonstrate the efficacy of culturally rooted and value-based interventions. In policy practice, their ability to extract the salutogenic value of ancestral teachings enables agency-level policy change to advance the inclusion of Indigenous knowledge in our formulations of wellness more widely. In research, they promote inclusiveness when weighing the types of reality that could exist and be retold about BMYOC and their communities.

Practice Implications

LCC and *El Joven Noble* enhance behavioural health practice among BYMOC by showing the utility of culturally rooted and value-based interventions in engaging BYMOC to a degree that conventional Western clinical interventions have not been documented to do. Their use of Indigenous mechicano indio core values transform the cultural identity and worldview of youth participants instead of simply reframing cognition of high-risk behaviour. By promoting intrinsic self-reform as such, LCC and El Joven Noble show that it is beneficial to promote an individual's connection to his cultural heritage via values-oriented teachings. By applying the mechicano indio knowledge system as a practical tool in soothing adolescence stress, LCC and El Joven Noble help practitioners rethink what knowledge systems could be included in practitioner training and service delivery.

Furthermore, LCC and El Joven Noble show that respecting the subjective personal and community-level reality of pain and fear in which BYMOC live could effectively move them toward wellness. BYMOC populations use different words and alternative perspectives to describe their subjective experience of the world; thus, mechicano indio knowledge and practices that acknowledge that subjectivity succeed in youth engagement because they facilitate greater understanding of Latinx, Chicano, Mexican American and Native youth.

Policy Implications

LCC and *El Joven Noble* widen options for agency-level policy change, particularly those impacting the design of behavioural health programming for BYMOC. That the mechicano indio knowledge system is not integrated into the Western medical model serves as an opportunity for agency-level policymaking to allow its wider use. LCC demonstrates how ancestral culture and values could be integrated into our formulations of wellness. Furthermore, by making it plausible that behavioural health programs based on Indigenous knowledge could be eligible for third-party health insurance reimbursement, we have an opportunity to redefine how we compensate for healthcare in the era of value-based versus fee-for-service-based care.

Research Implications

LCC has implications for evaluation research, particularly for Indigenous knowledge-based interventions. Conventional approaches to evaluation research are not reliably respectful of Indigenous communities and the original words of Latinx, Mexican American, Chicano, and Indigenous youth. Western evaluators' effort to aggregate responses into Western themes impose the supremacy of the Western approach to rationality, effacing non-Western worldviews.

   LCC promotes the use of a culturally rooted evaluation approach, enabling evaluation research to convey the reality experienced by Latinx, Mexican American, Chicano, and Indigenous youth more fully. It does so by describing and explaining that reality more specifically and in a much more balanced way – improving trust between researchers, evaluators, and communities. This, in turn, leads to more valid and meaningful data from our experience, thus, more effective service delivery models, for Latinx, Mexican American, Chicano, and Indigenous youth. By delivering access to subjective reality, LCC reduces the power imbalance between Western and non-Western views on what types of reality could exist (ontology) and the ways in which we could know reality (epistemology); therefore, in this chapter, we present the words of participants and public officials to show that evaluators who carefully listen are those who respectfully bridge voices of those that tell the stories and those that can make a difference.

Conclusion

In conclusion, LCC and El Joven Noble's use of Indigenous knowledge as the source for program theory and traditional rituals for process theory are effective practical uses of the therapeutic and salutogenic value of ancestral teachings. As culturally rooted and value-based interventions, LCC and El Joven Noble deepen intergenerational connectedness and an authentic cultural identity. They soothe adolescent stress and intergenerational trauma among BYMOC in the U.S. using ancestral mechicano indio teachings. They advance the inclusion of Indigenous knowledge in the conceptualization of health and wellbeing for BYMOC. Finally, LCC and El Joven Noble inform how we could heal BYMOC, particularly Latinx, Mexican American, Chicano, and Indigenous youth, who face the escalation of trauma-inducing anti-Latino, anti-immigrant racism, and catastrophic encounters with police and the justice system in the U.S.

References

Andrade, N., Ford, A. D., & Alvarez, C. (2020). Discrimination and Latino health: A systematic review of risk and resilience. *Hispanic Health Care International, 1540415320921489.*

Ardino, V. (2012). Offending behaviour: The role of trauma and PTSD. *European Journal of Psychotraumatology, 3.* https://doi.org/10.3402/ejpt.v3i0.18968

Bradshaw-Dieng, J., Valenzuela, J., & Ortiz, T. (2016). *Building the we; healing informed governing for racial equity in Salinas.* Race Forward, The Center for Racial Innovation.

Brave Heart, M., Chase, E., & J., Altschul, D.B. (2011). Historical trauma among indigenous peoples of the Americas: Concepts, research, and clinical considerations. *Journal of Psychoactive Drugs, 43*(4), 282–290. https://doi.org/10.1080/02791072.2011.628913

Cabrera, N., & Hennigar, A. (2019). The early home environment of Latino children: A research synthesis. *Child Trends.* https://www.childtrends.org/publications/the-early-home-environment-of-latino-children-a-research-synthesis

Centers for Disease Control (CDC). (2003). *Web-based injury statistics query and reporting system* (WISQARS). National Center for Injury Prevention and Control, Centers for Disease Control and Prevention.

Cerdeña, J. P., Rivera, L. M., & Spak, J. M. (2021). Intergenerational trauma in Latinxs: A scoping review. *Social Science & Medicine, 270*, 113662.

Coll, K., Freeman, B., Robertson, P., Cloud, E., Cloud Two Dog, E., & Two Dogs, R. (2012). Exploring Irish multigenerational trauma and its healing: Lessons from the Oglala Lakota (Sioux). *Advances in Applied Sociology, 2*, 95–101. https://doi.org/10.4236/aasoci.2012.22013

Dragomir, R. R., & Tadros, E. (2020). Exploring the impacts of racial disparity within the American juvenile justice system. *Juvenile & Family Court Journal, 71*, 61–73. https://doi.org/10.1111/jfcj.12165

Gibson, L. E., Holt, J. C., Fondacaro, K. M., Tang, T. S., Powell, T. A., & Turbitt, E. L. (1999). An examination of antecedent traumas and psychiatric comorbidity among male inmates with PTSD. *Journal of Traumatic Stress, 12*, 473–484.

Gonzales, N. A., Dumka, L. E., Millsap, R. E., Gottschall, A., McClain, D. B., Wong, J. J., Germán, M., Mauricio, A. M., Wheeler, L., Carpentier, F. D., & Kim, S. Y. (2012). Randomized trial of a broad preventive intervention for Mexican American adolescents. *Journal of Consulting and Clinical Psychology, 80*(1), 1–16. https://doi.org/10.1037/a0026063

Gonzales, N. A., Dumka, L. E., Millsap, R. E., Gottschall, A., McClain, D. B., Wong, J. J., Germán, M., Mauricio, A. M., Gonzalez, L. M., Mejia, Y., Kulish, A., Stein, G. L., Kiang, L., Fitzgerald, D., & Cavanaugh, A. (2020). Alternate approaches to coping in Latinx adolescents from immigrant families. *Journal of Adolescent Research, 37*(3), 353–377.

Graham, P. W., Yaros, A., Lowe, A., et al. (2017). Nurturing environments for boys and men of colour with trauma exposure. *Clinical Child Family Psychology Review, 20*, 105–116. https://doi.org/10.1007/s10567-017-0241-6

Hofstede, G., & Hofstede, G. J. (2010). *Cultures and organizations: Software of the mind, and cultures.* McGraw-Hill.

Isobel, S., Goodyear, M., Furness, T., & Foster, K. (2019). Preventing intergenerational trauma transmission: A critical interpretive synthesis. *Journal of Clinical Nursing, 28*(7–8), 1100–1113. https://doi.org/10.1111/jocn.14735

Jeffers, J. L. (2019). Justice is not blind: Disproportionate incarceration rate of people of colour. *Public Health, 34*(1), 113–121. https://doi.org/10.1080/19371918.2018.1562404

Jones, S. M., Bodie, G. D., & Hughes, S. D. (2019). The impact of mindfulness on empathy, active listening, and perceived provisions of emotional support. *Communication Research, 46*(6), 838–865. https://doi.org/10.1177/0093650215626983

Kluckhohn, F. R., & Strodtbeck, F. L. (1961). *Variations in value orientations.* Row, Peterson.

Koch, A., Brierley, C., Maslin, M., & Lewis, S. (2019). European colonization of the Americas killed 10 percent of world population and caused global cooling. *The Globe*, Retrieved from https://www.pri.org/stories/2019-01-31/european-colonization-americas-killed-10-percent-world-population-and-caused.

Kovera, M. B. (2019). Racial disparities in the criminal justice system: Prevalence, causes, and a search for solutions. *Journal of Social Issues, 75*(4), 1139–1164. https://doi.org/10.1111/josi.12355

Maschi, T., Bradley, C. A., & Morgen, K. (2008). Unraveling the link between trauma and delinquency: The mediating role of negative affect and delinquent peer exposure. *Youth Violence and Juvenile Justice, 6*(2), 136–157. https://doi.org/10.1177/1541204007305527

Orozco-Figueroa, A. (2021). The historical trauma and resilience of individuals of Mexican Ancestry in the United States: A scoping literature review and emerging conceptual framework. *Genealogy, 5*, 32. https://doi.org/10.3390/genealogy5020032

Prochaska, J. O., & Velicer, W. F. (1997). The transtheoretical model of health behaviour change. *American Journal of Health Promotion, 12*(1), 38–48. https://doi.org/10.4278/0890-1171-12.1.38

Santiago, C. D., Distel, L. M. L., Ros, A. M., et al. (2018). Mental health among Mexican-origin immigrant families: The roles of cumulative sociodemographic risk and immigrant-related stress. *Race & Social Problems, 10*(3), 235–247.

Spitzer, C., Dudeck, M., Liss, H., Orlob, S., Gillner, M., & Freyberger, H. J. (2001). Post-traumatic stress disorder in forensic inpatients. *Journal of Forensic Psychiatry, 12*(1), 63–77.

Tello, J. T. (2018). *Recovering your sacredness*. Sueños Publications.

Vanden WallBake, R. V. (2013). *Considering childhood trauma in the juvenile justice system: Guidance for attorneys and judges*. American Bar Association. https://www.americanbar.org/groups/public_interest/child_law/resources/child_law_practiceonline/child_law_practice/vol_32/november-2013/considering-childhood-trauma-in-the-juvenile-justice-system – gui/

Williams, M. T., Peña, A., & Mier-Chairez, J. (2017). Tools for assessing racism-related stress and trauma among Latinos. In L. Benuto (Ed.), *Toolkit for counseling Spanish-speaking clients* (pp. 71–95). Springer.

Wolff, N. L., & Shi, J. (2010). Trauma and incarcerated persons. In C. L. Scott (Ed.), *Handbook of correctional mental health* (pp. 277–320). American Psychiatric Publishing.

Chapter 11
Promoting Health and Wellbeing: Young Cook Islands Māori Men in New Zealand and the Cook Islands

Vili Nosa, Robbie Atatoa, Lisa Puloka, Malakai Ofanoa, Teuila Percival, and Debra de Silva

Introduction

Cook Islands Māori men have poor health outcomes whether they live in the Cook Islands or New Zealand. This includes lower life expectancies than other Pacific men. Modernisation, migration, and urbanisation have impacted dietary intake and physical activity, thus driving the obesity epidemic and the increase in NCDs in the Cook Islands. Imported foods such as rice, sugar, canned foods, and sugary drinks have replaced traditional foods such as taro, fish, fruits, and vegetables due to their increased affordability and accessibility. Consequently, more Cook Māori men are leading sedentary lifestyles, and fewer individuals are living off the land due to the physical demands of farming. When Cook Islands Maori men migrated to New Zealand for a better lifestyle, they also encountered a number of health-related issues: poor diet, obesity and a lack of physical activities. Access to low-cost fast-food outlets also contributed to the poor health of Cook Islands Māori men.

This chapter explores practical ways to improve the health and wellbeing of young Cook Islands Māori men using culturally grounded activities to promote health. We draw on research with Cook Islands Māori men between the ages of 18–25 years in both the Cook Islands and New Zealand.

V. Nosa (✉) · R. Atatoa · L. Puloka · M. Ofanoa · T. Percival · D. de Silva
Pacific Health Section, School of Population Health, The University of Auckland, Auckland, New Zealand
e-mail: v.nosa@auckland.ac.nz; robbieatatoa@xtra.co.nz; l.puloka@auckland.ac.nz; m.ofanoa@auckland.ac.nz; t.percival@auckland.ac.nz; debra@evidencecentre.com

© The Editor(s) (if applicable) and The Author(s), under exclusive license to Springer Nature Switzerland AG 2023
J. A. Smith et al. (eds.), *Health Promotion with Adolescent Boys and Young Men of Colour*, https://doi.org/10.1007/978-3-031-22174-3_11

The Cook Islands Health Profile

The Cook Islands is made up of 15 islands in the Pacific Ocean divided into two groups: the northern and the southern group. Over three-quarters of the population lives on the main island, Rarotonga. The main languages are English and Cook Islands Maori (mainly Rarotongan), with several different dialects.

As with other Pacific Islands, the main health issues affecting the population are non-communicable diseases such as cardiovascular diseases, cancers, chronic respiratory diseases, and Type 2 diabetes (Te Marae Ora Cook Islands Ministry of Health, 2015). The average life expectancy is around 71 years for men and 78 years for women (World Health Organization, 2011, 2017, 2018).

The Cook Islands National Strategy and Action Plan for Non-Communicable Diseases 2015–2019 has eight components including integrated activities, alcohol harm reduction, tobacco control, mental health and disability, food and nutrition, physical activities, national health system approach and monitoring, evaluation, and surveillance. One of the key priorities was to support better health outcomes for young people.

The government is the main provider of health care, including primary care and public health programmes (Te Marae Ora Cook Islands Ministry of Health, 2015); it is located on the island of Rarotonga and also provides services for the outer islands.

Health promotion activities include promoting healthy living at church services and youth groups, giving free health risk assessments at workplaces, and offering smoking cessation services on the main island of Rarotonga and 80% of the outer islands (Te Marae Ora Cook Islands Ministry of Health, 2015).

Very little research focuses on young Cook Islands Māori men. However, what we know about them is that they tend to have high rates of smoking and alcohol consumption, high cholesterol levels, high blood pressure, high rates of cardiovascular diseases and suicide rates. Their rates of consuming fruits and vegetables and participating in physical activities are low (Cook Island STEPS Survey 2013–2015 Fact Sheet).

Cook Islands Māori Men in New Zealand

The Cook Islands is one of New Zealand's three Pacific realm countries, which means it is independent but has close ties with New Zealand (Adam Smith International, 2015). Cook Islands people are New Zealand citizens and are entitled to use New Zealand healthcare services.

The Cook Islands population is the third-largest Pacific population in New Zealand, with around 80,500 members, half of whom are men, and whose median age is 21 years. About eight out of ten were born in New Zealand (83%). Nine out of ten speak English (94%) and one in five speak two or more languages (18%). This means that the majority of young Cook Islands Māori men in New Zealand do not speak Cook Islands Māori (Statistics New Zealand Census, 2018).

Research suggests that young Cook Islands Māori men living in New Zealand have poorer health when compared to other Pacific and non-Pacific men. They often have issues such as obesity, diabetes, cardiovascular diseases, depression, and low self-esteem (Natua, 2008). They have also been found to have higher rates of hospital admission and motor vehicle accidents (Health Partners Consulting Group, 2012).

Hearing from Cook Islands Māori Men

In New Zealand we interviewed a total of 8 Cook Islands Māori men aged between 18–25 years old. We hired a Cook Islands research assistant who was able to interview the men in English and Cook Islands Maori. The interviews were done in the Tokoroa region, Waikato, as this was where the research assistant was based. The interviews took place at a time and venue convenient to the participants, mostly food malls, community venues, and men's homes. Most of them had a secondary school and tertiary qualification. Most of them were employed, married, and belong to a religious denomination. To acknowledge participants' time, we gave each one a $50 food voucher after the interview.

We also interviewed a total of 9 Cook Islands men aged between 18–25 years old living in the Cook Islands. For consistency, the interviews were undertaken by the same Cook Islands researcher that did the interviews in New Zealand. Due to time and travel limitations, all the participants were interviewed on the main island of Rarotonga. While most of the men were born in the Cook Islands, a few were born overseas but had returned to the Cook Islands for family reasons and employment opportunities. Some of them had completed a secondary school and tertiary qualification; some did not have a qualification. Most of them worked in the public and private sector. Most of them were married and belonged to a church. $50 cash was provided to the men to thank them for their participation in the research.

The key questions in the interviews consisted of the definition of a Niuean man; definition of health; self-rated health; health beliefs and practices; knowledge and use of healthcare services; cultural issues around health; perceived barriers to accessing healthcare services; and potential healthcare services. Three of the authors independently read the transcripts to identify the major key themes. A general inductive thematic analysis consisted of eliciting key themes that were repeated and thereby evident in the data. (Thomas, 2006). We received ethics approval from the University of Auckland Human Subjects Committee Ref. 020659 and the Cook Islands Research Committee.

Exploring Men's Health Values

Health Beliefs and Behaviours

Many of the participants defined the concept of health in terms of being able to stay physically fit by being active and eating healthy foods. There was a difference here between young men in the Cook Islands and in New Zealand. Those in the Cook Islands thought that their traditional foods were healthy, and that the introduction of Western foods and behaviours was causing issues:

> When you think about health you think mostly about the old people, when we were living mostly on natural foods. If you look at the old pictures, you see how healthy and how strong the men were before. When other foods were introduced, you can see the changes of the body types, as people got bigger and obese [to] where you can't even walk properly now. – *Man in the Cook Islands 25 years*

> In the years before when nana and papa were hunters and gatherers, there was no freezer. We were out there on the reef or on the taro patch. Eating the herbs and the berries and things like that. Today most of us are going to takeaways. We are no longer walking the reef anymore. – *Man in the Cook Islands 24 years*

Young men in New Zealand stated that good physical health included exercise and healthy eating, but they did not usually reference changes to the diet. However, some acknowledged that overeating traditional food could be associated with health issues:

> We eat too much of our traditional food which has a lot of coconut cream, fatty products. – *Man in New Zealand 20 years*

In New Zealand young Cook Islands Maori men were more likely to take a holistic view of health:

> Health to me would be all aspects of health, so mental wellbeing especially, but also being physically healthy. And health is just all aspects of your life that contribute to it. How well we interact with others and how well we hold our families together. – *Man in New Zealand 21 years*

Most of the men spoke about risk factors such as being overweight, limited physical activity, obesity, diabetes, gout and alcohol use:

> Probably our eating, our diets… mainly that. Being overweight. – *Man in the Cook Islands 20 years*

> Well, aside from like the norm for us Cook Island men with our eating habits – well, more like overeating habits – is uh, our lack of time we spend actually being physical – *Man in New Zealand 19 years*

> Like gout, diabetes, obesity is a problem. – *Man in New Zealand 21 years*

> I have a family that can drink every day. It becomes a habit. I know it's a major problem to their health. It's one of the biggest issues we do have here in the Cook Islands. – *Man in the Cook Islands 19 years*

Using Healthcare Services

Young men in New Zealand and the Cook Islands had very similar opinions about using healthcare services. Men tried to avoid using health services whenever possible. If men felt unwell, they said they would usually wait it out until they got better, or they would self-medicate with medicines such as Panadol. Men said they would only seek medical treatment if their health issues got worse or if they were encouraged by family members:

> For me, I usually see the doctor if I am really sick. I try hold off as much as I can. – *Man in the Cook Islands 19 years*

> If it gets worse, well, then maybe I'll go. My mum tells me to go to the doctors when I am really sick. My mum always pushes me to go. – *Man in New Zealand 18 years*

Young men reported that they avoided visiting health services because they were stubborn, and it was a matter of pride. However, their comments indicated that many young men thought that not using health services was part of being a Cook Islander, so this avoidant behaviour is thought to be culturally grounded:

> A lot of our Cook Islands men are too proud to go the doctors… They don't wanna [want to] in that sort of environment just because they're too proud. – *Man in the Cook Islands 22 years*

> As Cook Islanders you don't go to the doctors. You get told to harden up, and I think beliefs like that are there to impress other people, which is just a cultural thing they were brought up with. Their parents have told them harden up… it's almost like a negative thing to go and see a doctor. – *Man in New Zealand 25 years*

> I think they're too shy or too – what's the word – ashamed. Too ashamed and too scared, I would say. I think it's just that fear of going to see a doctor or just even go for a free check-up. I think that's the common cultural issue around it, being ashamed and too scared. – *Man in the Cook Islands 24 years*

Promoting Health and Wellbeing

We asked what would encourage young men to use health services or take part in health promotion activities or healthy behaviours. In both New Zealand and the Cook Islands, most men said they would feel more comfortable with a Cook Islands healthcare provider. The men thought that just having someone from the same background to speak with would be motivational:

> A lot more people will feel more comfortable with someone from their own culture running a health clinic. I think especially in our older generation where they might be too shy to come in and stuff like that but if they see someone from the islands or someone of Cook Island descent that's reassuring. – *Man in New Zealand 23 years*

The men thought that it would be useful to have multiple services offered in one place. They said it was off-putting to have to travel to multiple locations to access different services:

> Services that are available, because there are parts where some of us Cook Island men need to go to physio, you know. The doctor will tell you to go here, there, and everywhere but if they got all the services in one place,… then everything's there, you know. – *Man in New Zealand 23 years*

As transport was a barrier in both New Zealand and the Cook Islands, men in both countries suggested that mobile health clinics or transport services to help people get to healthcare providers would increase usage in the Cook Islands community:

> Maybe a delivery and pickup service so Cook Islands men can get to the health clinics. This was a barrier for me to get to the doctors. This would also help to get other family members to the clinic as well. – *Man in the Cook Islands 19 years*

Young men said there was a need to provide health education to raise awareness amongst Cook Island men about making healthy choices and the availability of healthcare services. They also suggested healthy eating and fitness programmes. They wanted practical classes to help them stay active and learn about healthy eating:

> Probably like more education and the nutrition side of things so we know what's bad for us and what's good for us. – *Man in the Cook Islands 19 years*

> Implement a cooking programme for the men so they understand about healthy eating… with things like taking them shopping, making them read food labels… how much sugar in this, how much fat in that, what is good for you and what is bad for you. Also have an exercise programme for the men. – *Man in the Cook Islands 25 years*

> I think we need like a fitness group, you know, a men's-only fitness group where you can train at your own level at your own pace. – *Man in the Cook Islands 19 years*

Discussion

Young Cook Islands Māori men in New Zealand and the Cook Islands have poor and inequitable health outcomes and demonstrate a reluctance to seek help. However, our research suggests that health promotion activities could make inroads if they are culturally grounded, well-framed, and proactive. For example, the work by the National Hauora Coalition et al. (2020) notes that the use of developing health promotion strategies outlined the concept of "by Pacific, for Pacific," which means health promotion strategies need to be designed and led by Pacific people. Such efforts should include early education, be family-based and utilize strong, direct messaging. Glover et al. (2019) also notes that Pacific communities need to develop health promotion programmes that are culturally appropriate and suitable for Pacific communities. Therefore, Cook Islands Māori men and Cook Islands health promoters need to be at the forefront of developing health promotion messages for strategies targeting Cook Islands young men to be effective. On the other hand, international authors (Smith et al., 2020; Kaholokula et al., 2018, Manson 2020; Walters et al., 2020) also find that culturally appropriate strategies for Indigenous populations are effective and useful in promoting better health outcomes.

The men in this study spoke about health education workshops, such as eating and fitness programmes, as a key avenue for providing better awareness and improving health outcomes. Ryan et al. (2019) also found that holding health education workshops specifically designed for and targeted to Pacific communities improves health outcomes for Pacific people.

The men in this research project mentioned how influential their family members were in their seeking medical care. This parallels Smith et al.'s (2020) examination of young Aboriginal and Torres Strait Islanders males in Australia, which showed that family are critical to the way they conceptualise health and seek health care advice. What our study highlights is the potential for targeting health promotion activities at the family level, rather than solely at the level of the individual.

Some of the men mentioned a lack of transport to the clinics as as a key barrier for not attending health services. The work of the Health Quality & Safety Commission (2021) also supports the finding that transport was a barrier for Pacific people to attend medical clinics. Providing mobile clinics and home doctor visits may be viable options for better health outcomes for these men, and would also encourage other family members to attend health clinics.

The World Health Organisation surveys health in countries similar to the Cook Islands, and suggests that health promotion should focus on promoting local foods, establishing physical activity-friendly environments, building sustainable government funding and health infrastructures, and integrating disease prevention and control into the policies and strategies of relevant government agencies. They also recommend improving health promotion campaigns and increasing public awareness on the importance of regularly screening blood pressure, blood cholesterol and blood sugar levels (World Health Organization, 2017, 2018). This is a reminder that health promotion needs to take place at multiple levels and requires funding and infrastructure that targets population health, as well as interventions that target individuals. Improving health equity access and providing better support for the social determinants of health will enable improved health outcomes. For instance, poor health literacy is a known factor for why Pacific people do not access primary health care services. Pio & Nosa's (2020) study on the health literacy of Samoan mothers and their experiences with health professionals found a need for user-friendly resources, such as visually accessible charts and diagrams, interactive activities and written information provided in both Samoan and English. However, while useful, these recommendations are relatively generic. Moving towards more specifics, our research suggests that young men in both New Zealand and the Cook Islands are interested in sharing their ideas and getting involved in developing health promotion initiatives.

The Pu Ara model is an example of health promotion developed to empower adolescents in the Cook Islands to improve their health and wellbeing. The model, which is built on a strengths-based approach, emphasises the importance of listening to young people. It demonstrates that health promotion activities must target the overall community, be inclusive and focus on participation (Herman, 2013). Rather than assuming that existing healthcare approaches and services will be accepted, service providers must centre Young Cook Islands men in the process of developing health promotion activities. This aligns with other research suggesting that ethnic-specific models of health promotion improve health outcomes when designed by indigenous or minority ethnic groups and built by the community in a bottom-up approach. (Koroigasagasa & Nosa, 2021).

We recommend that health promotion for Young Cook Islands Māori *men living in New Zealand* focus on:

- Health education programmes to provide practical advice about how to make healthy lifestyle changes. Young men seem to know that it would be useful to make changes, but they say they do not have knowledge about how to break habits or what foods are good for them. Churches, sports groups, and community groups could all be vehicles for promoting and hosting such programmes, as men said they liked to combine social and health activities. (Hopoi & Nosa, 2020).
- Raising awareness about the range of (free) services available. Men were reluctant to visit doctors, but there are many other healthcare and support services available, including church groups and community groups. A communications campaign could raise awareness via Cook Islands radio programmes and the Cook Islands Health Network Association (NZ), which advocates and represents the healthcare interests of Cook Islands people in New Zealand.
- Studying the feasibility of a Cook Islands health provider, so that men can communicate in their own language or with people from their own cultural background. This would provide a safe place for men to talk to male health professionals. Such a study should also investigate whether to support a mobile clinic to visit communities where Cook Islands men live, since transport is often a barrier. (Ryan et al., 2019).

We recommend that health promotion for Young Cook Islands Māori men *living in the Cook Islands* focus on:

- Providing healthy eating and fitness programmes within the community, including workshops suitable for young men. These could be run in partnership between government health services and churches, village groups and local sports teams to help to normalise and promote healthy lifestyles.
- Extending health education programmes to cover health issues affecting men such as prostate cancer, diabetes, and alcohol awareness. Our interviews suggest that men are looking for information that is appropriate and easy to understand. Social media, technology and radio could help to spread messages as these are popular in the Cook Islands. (Ringi et al., 2021).
- Developing initiatives to recruit young, male Cook Islands health professionals from overseas to return to work in the Cook Islands, as the health workforce there is very limited.
- Considering home visits by health professionals to communicate with the 'hard to reach' men and those less likely to visit services when they are unwell. This is more likely to affect older men, but may also benefit younger men who do not have access to transportation.

Conclusion

There is a growing population of young Cook Islands men in both the Islands and New Zealand. This is largely a youthful population, but these men suffer from or are at risk of a range of preventable, non-communicable diseases. Based on feedback from young men, there are a variety of strategies that can help men to take ownership of developing healthy positive lives. There is already some good work happening in the Cook Islands including research (Herman, 2013; Te Marae Ora Cook Islands Ministry of Health, 2015), so some health promotion messages and activities may also be relevant in New Zealand. Families may be interested in taking part in effective health promotion programmes that have worked or been implemented in the Cook Islands.

References

Adam Smith International. (2015). *Evaluation of the Cook Islands Country Programme*. Retrieved from https://www.mfat.govt.nz/assets/Aid-Prog-docs/Evaluations/2015/Dec-2015/Evaluation-CPE-Cook-Islands-Report-Final-Dec2015.pdf

Cook Island STEPS Survey 2013–2015 Fact Sheet. Retrieved from https://www.who.int/publications/m/item/2013-2015-steps-fact-sheet-cook-islands

Glover M., Wong S. F., Fa'alili-Fidow J., Derraik J. G. B., Taylor R. W., Morton S. M. B., Tautolo E. S., Cutfield W. S. (2019). Ranked importance of childhood obesity determinants: parents' views across ethnicities in New Zealand. *Nutrients, 11*(9):2145. https://doi.org/10.3390/nu11092145. PMID: 31500336; PMCID: PMC6769712.

Health Partners Consulting Group. (2012). *Metro-Auckland Pacific population health profile*. Health Partners Consulting Group.

Health Quality & Safety Commission. (2021). *Bula Sautu – A window on quality 2021: Pacific health in the year of COVID-19*. Health Quality & Safety Commission.

Herman, N. (2013). *Investing in our young people: Akaupokotuanga I Ta Tatou Mapu No Te Au Tuatau Ki Mua* (Unpublished PhD thesis, University of Auckland, New Zealand).

Hopoi, N., & Nosa, V. (2020). A qualitative study of the role of Samoan Church Ministers in health literacy messages and health promotion in Auckland, New Zealand. *Australian & New Zealand Journal of Public Health, 44*, 404–409. https://doi.org/10.1111/1753-6405.13027

Kaholokula, K., Townsend, C., Look, M., Delafield, R., & Sinclair, K. (2018). Culturally responsive approaches to health promotion for Native Hawaiians and Pacific Islanders. *Annals of Human Biology, 45*(3), 243–263. https://doi.org/10.1080/03014460.2018.1465593

Koroigasagasa, T., & Nosa, V. (2021). A systematic review of diabetes mellitus in Fiji. *Global Scientific Journal, 9*(7), 1903–1916.

Manson, S. (2020). The role of culture in effective intervention design, implementation, and research: Its universal importance. *Prevention Science, 21*(Suppl 1), 93–97. https://doi.org/10.1007/s11121-019-01065-7

Natua, J. (2008). *A case study of Cook Island men in Tokoroa, New Zealand* (Unpublished master's thesis in Public Health). University of Auckland, Auckland.

Pio, F., & Nosa, V. (2020). Health literacy of Samoan mothers and their experiences with health professionals. *Journal of Primary Health Care, 12*, 57–63.

Ringi, T., Herman, J., Tairi, M., Dobson, R., Nosa, V., Whittaker, R., & McCool, J. (2021). *Takore i te Kai Ava'ava,* a cessation programme adapted for the Cook Islands: Indicators of potential for tobacco control. *Asia Pacific Journal of Public Health, 33*(6–7), 714–720. https://doi.org/10.1177/10105395211036267

Ryan, D., Grey, C., & Mischewski, B. (2019). *Tofa saili: A review of evidence about health equity for Pacific peoples in New Zealand*. Pacific Perspectives, Ltd.,

The National Hauora Coalition; Anderson, A., Brown, R., Wheeler, J., Jansen, R. (2020). Pacific Fono: a community based initiative to improve rheumatic fever service delivery for Pacific Peoples in South Auckland. *J Prim Health Care, 12*(4):384–390. https://doi.org/10.1071/HC20022

Smith, J. A., Merlino, A., Christie, B., Adams, M., Bonson, J., Osborne, R., Judd, B., Drummond, M., Aanundsen, D., & Fleay, J. (2020). 'Dudes are meant to be tough as nails': The complex nexus between masculinities, culture and health literacy from the perspective of young Aboriginal and Torres Strait Islander males – Implications for policy and practice. *American Journal of Men's Health, 14*(3), 1–17.

Statistics New Zealand. (2018). *Cook Islands Maori ethnic group*. https://www.stats.govt.nz/tools/2018-census-ethnic-group-summaries/cook-islands-maori

Te Marae Ora Cook Islands Ministry of Health. (2015). *Cook Islands national strategy and action plan for non-communicable diseases 2015–2019*. Te Marae Ora Cook Islands Ministry of Health.

Thomas, D. R. (2006). A general inductive approach for analyzing qualitative evaluation data. *American Journal of Evaluation, 27*(2), 237–246.

Walters, K. L., Johnson-Jennings, M., Stroud, S., et al. (2020). Growing from our roots: Strategies for developing culturally grounded health promotion interventions in American Indian, Alaska Native, and Native Hawaiian Communities. *Prevention Science, 21*(Suppl 1), 54–64. https://doi.org/10.1007/s11121-018-0952-z

World Health Organization. (2011). *Cook Islands NCD risk factors STEPS report*. WHO Western Pacific Region. https://www.health.gov.ck/wp-content/uploads/2020/06/Cook-Islands-STEPS-Report-2013-2015.pdf

World Health Organization. (2017). *WHO country cooperation strategy 2018–2022: Pacific Island Countries and Areas*. WHO Regional Office for the Western Pacific.

World Health Organization. (2018). *Country corporation strategy at a glance*. https://www.who.int/publications/i/item/WHO-CCU-18.02-Cook-Islands

Chapter 12
Promoting Cultural Identity as a Form of Health Promotion for New Zealand-Born Niue Men in Aotearoa (New Zealand)

Vili Nosa, Kava Fuavao, Lisa Puloka, Malakai Ofanoa, Teuila Percival, and Debra de Silva

Introduction

Young Pacific men in Aotearoa (New Zealand) and in the Pacific Islands suffer from high rates of obesity, diabetes, smoking, problem drinking, high blood pressure, disability, a range of chronic conditions, and early death. They also see older male relatives suffer the devastating effects of these conditions, which are often preventable but systemic in Niue communities.

Promoting health and wellbeing for Niue men can improve younger men's physical and mental health and save lives. However, many health promotion strategies fail because they are not grounded in the beliefs and values of local communities. They are "done to" people rather than built with and for them. They do not account for differences between older and younger men or target younger men to champion new ways of thinking and acting.

In this chapter we show how understanding cultural identity and "being a Niue man" is essential for promoting health and wellbeing amongst young Niue men in Aotearoa. We argue that health promotion that appreciates and embeds Niue culture is likely to be more successful than the "standardised" Western approaches currently available. This chapter explores the views and perceptions of New Zealand-born Niue men between 16–25 years old.

V. Nosa (✉) · K. Fuavao · L. Puloka · M. Ofanoa · T. Percival · D. de Silva
Pacific Health Unit, School of Population Health, The University of Auckland, Auckland, New Zealand
e-mail: v.nosa@auckland.ac.nz; kfua002@aucklanduni.ac.nz; l.puloka@auckland.ac.nz; m.ofanoa@auckland.ac.nz; t.percival@auckland.ac.nz; debra@evidencecentre.com

183

Setting the Scene – Niue Men in Aotearoa

There are 381,642 Pacific people who call Aotearoa home, made up of 13 different Pacific ethnic groups. The Niue population are the fourth-largest Pacific community in Aotearoa, with 30,867 Niuean people living in Aotearoa. In fact, about 15 times more Niue people live in Aotearoa than on the island of Niue. (Statistics New Zealand, 2018). Niue is one of the world's smallest independent island nations (260 square km). Located between Tonga and the Cook Islands approximately 2100 km northeast of New Zealand, Niue is one of the largest raised coral atolls in the world.

Niue has a special relationship with Aotearoa. Niue people are citizens of Aotearoa and can move freely between the countries for employment, educational opportunities and what many perceive to be a better lifestyle (Nosa, 2020). This is possible because of a unique historical relationship: Niue became a British protectorate in 1900 and was annexed by Aotearoa in 1901. In 1974 the people of Niue adopted a constitution providing for full self-government in free association with Aotearoa. (McDonald, 2018).

About 15,000 Niue men live in Aotearoa. Most Niue people in Aotearoa were born there (83%) or have lived there for over 20 years (76%). As of the last census, the median age was about 22 years, and the median income was about $24,000 – a relatively low wage by local standards. Almost all Niue people in Aotearoa speak English as their main language (95%), with just one in five speaking two languages (21%) (Statistics New Zealand, 2018).

Very little research has been conducted about the health of Niue people in Aotearoa. Niue people's life expectancy is significantly lower than the national average and the average for Pacific people in Aotearoa. The top five causes of death are largely preventable diseases, such as ischaemic heart disease, diabetes, stroke, and chronic obstructive respiratory diseases. (Health Partners Consulting Group, 2012; Novak, 2007). Though the information available paints a bleak picture, it also showcases the potential benefits of promoting health and wellbeing.

Compared to the total population and the Pacific population of Aotearoa, Niue men have higher rates of hospital admission, diabetes-related operations, rheumatic fever, skin disorders, epilepsy, dementia, mental illness, psychosis, stroke, cataract surgery, alcohol, and cancer rates (Health Partners Consulting Group, 2012). Around 11% of Niue men in Aotearoa smoke; the same proportion as for Niue women (Statistics New Zealand, 2018).

This evidence suggests that while many of the young Niue men in Aotearoa have lived all or most of their lives in Aotearoa, they do not speak Niuean fluently. They see the effects of poor health in their community and amongst close relatives and may suffer from chronic conditions themselves. Health promotion could make a big difference to the lives and wellbeing of young Niuean men. Yet anecdotal evidence suggests that younger Niue men do not visit health services or take part in health promotion activities.

Listening to Niue Men

We interviewed 11 men in Aotearoa aged between 16–25 years, all of whom were born in New Zealand. Half worked in manufacturing or labour jobs, a quarter had an office job, and a quarter were at secondary school or a tertiary institution. Most of them were religious and belonged to a church.

We hired a young male Pacific research assistant based in the Auckland region to conduct interviews there. We conducted face-to-face interviews in English using a semi-structured schedule. The interviews took place in the men's homes, community venues or other venues named by the participants. The research assistant conducted all of the interviews for consistency, spending some time to build rapport with each interviewee before formally beginning the interview. With participants' consent, each interview was audio recorded and transcribed. The interview guide was tested before beginning the study and the research team reviewed the transcripts of initial interviews to validate the approach and questions. A NZ$50-dollar gift voucher incentive was provided to the participants to acknowledge their time in participating in this research.

The key questions in the interviews consisted of the definition of a Niuean man; definition of health; self-rated health; health beliefs and practices; knowledge and use of healthcare services; cultural issues around health; perceived barriers to accessing healthcare services; and potential healthcare services. Three of the authors read the transcripts to identify the key themes. (Thomas, 2006).

A general inductive approach was used to analyse the interview data, to allow findings to emerge from frequent or dominant themes expressed there. Each transcript was read systematically and multiple times by the authors to identify and code consistent themes. Three authors independently extracted themes by counting the number of occurrences. A fourth researcher cross-checked the themes to align them with our research aims. Illustrative quotes were drawn out to showcase the richness of the responses. Ethics approval was from the University of Auckland Human Subjects Committee Ref. 020659.

Building Young Men's Values into Health Promotion

We summarise some of the feedback here to show how young men's values and cultural identity were linked to their health attitudes and behaviours.

Being a Niuean Man

All of the men held strong views about what it means to be a Niue man, even those still at school. The components of being a Niuean man included:

- Taking pride in the Niuean culture, knowing your roots and actively taking part in cultural activities, such as trying to speak or understand the Niuean language and engaging in cultural practices such as hair cutting ceremonies
- Focusing on family and community
- Taking on challenges
- Christian beliefs
- Reciprocity, being generous and giving to the family and others:

> A Niue man is somebody who is confident, strong in their beliefs…like using the language and maybe some traditional practices, like can do you do a *umu* or can you recite many verses from the bible or in Niuean? – *Niue man 25 years*

> There's one thing I know with Niueans: there's always this reciprocal approach… we often give; and if we don't have enough to give, we still give. – *Niue man 23 years*

Health Beliefs and Behaviours

Participants told us that health was about maintaining balance and being happy. Most thought that they were in good health, even though some had diabetes, alcohol issues or perhaps ate less healthily than they could:

> It's not too bad, it's just my eating and stuff and my proportions are bigger. – *Niue man 21 years*

> I think I'm pretty good. I don't have any issues in regard to how I can walk; I can drive, I can see well with my glasses, you know, so I can do all those everyday things. – *Niue man 24 years*

There was also an element of wanting to be self-sufficient and look after oneself rather than needing to ask for help. This was just as prevalent in younger men, who prioritised an ability to look after themselves:

> Definition of health is having the ability to kind of look after yourself in whatever terms it may be; and try to maintain a healthy lifestyle; and exercising; eating appropriately; and be looked after mentally and physically. – *Nue man 22 years*

Given this focus on looking after yourself, it is perhaps unsurprising that Niue men emphasised ways of self-medicating. For young men this included over-the-counter painkillers to help them feel better. As one participant stated that he usually takes a Panadol or Nurofen. When further questioned on whether Panadol is the cure for everything, he stated:

> That's one thing, aye, in the household man, there's always paracetamol somewhere in the house. – *Niue man 19 years*

Another said:

> It's always the go-to thing: Panadol, or try the natural stuff when you got the flu you have lemon drinks… – *Niue man 18 years*

Using Healthcare Services

The young men said they had good knowledge of the healthcare services available to them in Aotearoa. They indicated that if a medical condition did not improve over time, going to health services was a last resort. The men often relied on the views of older family members, particularly if parents or aunties used an extended "wait and watch" approach:

> When it starts to get worse then my family will take me. They'll see how it turns out and once they see it gets bad, they'll take me to the doctors. – *Niue man 22 years*

> When I become sick, the first person I would go to will be the person closest to me to help me. Like for example, if I am worried, the first person I will ring is my wife. Then, only secondary to that will be going to see the doctor, but only if it gets much worse. – *Niue man 24 years*

Most of the young men we spoke with said that family input would be key in influencing their health behaviours and encouraging them to seek help from health services. This suggests that health promotion messages targeting women and wider families may filter through to Niue men.

> One way of getting men to the doctor is their family. Their wife or their children. I know women are very good supporters of their husband and encouraging their husband to go to their doctor… – *Niue man 23 years*

> I think my mum tries [to] influence me in regard to the immunisation, how important it is. How I perceive immunisation is how she sees it. – *Niue man 19 years*

Cultural Issues Affecting Health and Healthcare

Young men suggested that cultural issues influenced their health and healthcare. In our conversations, even younger men born in Aotearoa who did not speak Niuean still felt a strong sense of cultural identity and pride. While we see this as positive, it also had negative impacts on how men viewed health and healthcare. Participants said that they often would not visit a doctor due to pride or stubbornness. They perceived that a real Niue man would not ask for help if they became ill:

> I think it's to do with pride and being ashamed. They don't want to know that they are sick. They don't want other people to know that there's a sick person. – *Niue man 25 years*

Another cultural issue affecting Niue men was the importance of food in the Niue culture. Participants said that they knew Niue traditional foods can be fatty, but they were expected to eat a lot to show their appreciation. The gifting of food also plays a role in the cultural value of reciprocity. Taking part in cultural activities and traditions was important to men's conceptualisation of masculinity. Sometimes eating fatty or unhealthy foods contributed to men's identity as Niue men, even if the result over time was excess weight, high blood pressure or other health conditions:

> It's the eating. Real fatty foods like that [are] just bad for the health. When we have our Niue functions and big events, we usually have pigs, coconut cream in our taros and fatty corn beef and stuff like that. It is just part of who we are. – *Niue man 20 years*

Cost was another significant barrier to accessing healthcare services:

> Going to the doctor's is costly and expensive to pay. They can be quite expensive. – *Niue man 19 years*

A related barrier to using healthcare services was a perceived lack of time. Men often worked long hours to contribute income to their families. They said that healthcare services were not easily accessible outside their working hours:

> A lot of times I don't go and see a doctor because I need to be at work to support the family or there's no money. – *Niue man 24 years*

Promoting Health and Wellbeing

Cultural values and perceptions amongst Niue men can be harnessed to promote and support community wellbeing. Men were passionate about the potential for building health and wellbeing services that appealed to them and their communities. They said they would like to see Niue role models promote positive health messages via TV advertisements or social media:

> They could do that on the TV advertisement you know. Having a Niue role model would bring back that positive health message. – *Niue man 23 years*

Another suggestion was having workshops to raise awareness amongst Niue men about how to have a healthy lifestyle while maintaining their cultural beliefs and norms. Men suggested that this could provide a safe place to freely talk about health concerns. Participants suggested community venues, churches, or sports centres to make workshops more inviting and accessible. They also wanted to mix older and younger Niue men, as part of learning about and maintaining their cultural identity:

> Educate Niuean men by having workshops. The health workshops should have group discussions or health talks in the church groups about health issues that affect Niue men. – *Niue man 24 years*

> There should be space for them to sit down and actually talk about themselves. We need to have these workshops... just sit down and have a good conversation about looking after yourself. – *Niue man 25 years*

Discussion

This chapter has discussed how Niue cultural identity had a significant impact on how men thought about health and healthcare. The use of cultural identity in strengths-based health promotion can be an effective approach for better health outcomes for younger Niue men. For example, for younger Niue men the use of cultural elements – such as Niue manhood – is linked to healthy diet and physical activity, pointing the way forward for better messages for promoting health. Traditional stereotypes of cultured masculinity, which are core to Niue men's identity, may also be useful and acceptable. Understanding this could help in developing health promotion messages and activities. Research by The National Hauora Coalition et al. (2020) and Harding et al. (2021) found that building culturally appropriate strategies that incorporated cultural leaders for Pacific and indigenous populations helps improve health disparities for minority ethnic groups.

Family members can also assist in health promotion for younger Niue men. As we have noted, family members were a key factor influencing Niue men in accessing medical services. As an individual approach may not always be the most effective mode for health promotion messages because Niuean families act as collective units, targeting health promotional activities at the family level offers a productive way to achieve better health outcomes for young Niue men. These findings are similar to a recent study by Smith et al. (2020) whereby families played an important part in medical advice and support for Aboriginal and Torres Strait Islander men.

Participants also mentioned that Niue role models could act as a health promotion tool for providing positive health promotion messages. This in turn would provide a sense of inclusiveness for Niue men to get the health support they need. Hopoi & Nosa (2020) note in their study that role models like Samoan church ministers are a key source of positive health promotion messages within their congregations.

Younger Niue men liked the idea of having health workshops just for Niue men. Such workshops would provide a safe space for Niue men to share health information specifically applicable to men, like information about prostate cancer. These workshops could be more interactive and informative. These findings replicate the findings for the study about Niue men's perceptions of health and health services on the Island of Niue by Nosa et al. (2020). The men in that study were keen to have workshops that could educate Niue men on healthier lifestyles.

Anecdotally, Niue men are less likely than Niue women and the broader Aotearoa population to visit health services when they feel unwell. Our participants suggested that seeking help might not be perceived as a manly thing to do. There may be merit in considering how competitions and contests could help overcome those barriers and biases. For example, studies by Glover et al. (2014, 2015) found that competing for prizes was a good incentive for quitting smoking for Maori women. This might be a good idea to encourage younger Niue men's participation in health promotion activities, as well.

There are around 15,000 Niuean men in Aotearoa. Of this number, Niue men aged between 15–25 years represent 19%. (Statistics New Zealand, 2018). As the physical and mental health conditions afflicting Niue men are largely preventable and treatable, appropriate health promotion could have a major impact in saving lives, keeping families together and avoiding unnecessary emotional turmoil.

Appropriate health promotion need not require extensive new resources. It is about using the information, funding and skills already available in ways that place the local populations and individuals at the heart of the conversation, listening to their needs, fears and dreams. For example:

- To young Niue men in Aotearoa, being a Niue man was about taking pride and actively participating in cultural practices, attending church, and providing for their family. Health was defined as maintaining balance between physical, mental, emotional, and spiritual health. Health services and promoters could work with the Niue community to build on these values.
- Awareness-raising sessions and basic health services could be offered on church premises.
- Public health messaging using Niue or Pacific Island role models would catch people's attention as it is unusual, and has the potential to engage local men.
- Messaging could also emphasise the importance of staying well and accessing healthcare services promptly as a way of serving the family and church community.
- Since some young Niue men see being sick as a sign of weakness, we need to reframe messages to express that seeking healthcare and maintaining health is a sign of strength, ensuring that Niue men can live long and healthy lives and continue to support their families.

Conclusion

In conclusion, we learned much from what men told us about the kinds of health promotion messages and services that would appeal to them. They were not averse to taking care of themselves but needed to see this as benefitting their families and communities. Most importantly, we found that they held strong views about what it means to be a Niuean man — and that these views significantly impacted their health behaviours. If services can acknowledge and address these values, health promotion activities would likely be better received.

For young Niue men in Aotearoa, cultural identity is a significant part of who they are and how they view health and healthcare. Using words that are meaningful in a Niue context, centring health promotion messages around family and community, and having Niue people involved in delivering messages will all be key to whether young Niue men in Aotearoa can break cycles of poverty and health inequality to become champions for health and wellbeing in their communities.

References

Glover, M., Kira, A., Gentles, D., et al. (2014). The WERO group stop smoking competition: Main outcomes of a pre- and post- study. *BMC Public Health, 14*, 599.

Glover, M., Kira, A., Walker, N., et al. (2015). Using incentives to encourage smoking abstinence among pregnant indigenous women? A feasibility study. *Maternal and Child Health Journal, 19*(6), 1393–1399.

Harding, T., Oetzel, J. G., Foote, J., & Hepi, M. (2021). Perceptions of co-designing health promotion interventions with indigenous communities in New Zealand. *Health Promotion International., 36*(4), 964–975.

Health Partners Consulting Group. (2012). *Metro-Auckland Pacific population health profile*. HPCG.

Hopoi, N., & Nosa, V. (2020). A qualitative study of the role of Samoan church ministers in health literacy messages and health promotion in Auckland, New Zealand. *Australia and New Zealand Journal of Public Health, 44*, 404–409.

McDonald, C. (2018). *Decolonisation and free association: The relationships of the Cook Islands and Niue with New Zealand.* Unpublished PhD thesis. Victoria: University of Wellington, New Zealand.

New Zealand Statistics. (2018). Niuean ethnic group. https://www.stats.govt.nz/tools/2018-census-ethnic-group-summaries/niuean

Nosa, V., Fuavao, K., & de Silva, D. (2020). Men's perception of health and health services on the island of Niue: A qualitative study. *Journal of Global Health Reports, 4*, e2020054.

Novak, B. (2007). *Ethnic-specific health needs assessment for pacific people in counties Manukau.* Manukau City: Counties Manukau District health board.

Smith, J. A., Merlino, A., Christie, B., Adams, M., et al. (2020). 'Dudes are meant to be tough as nails': The complex nexus between masculinities, culture and health literacy from the perspective of young aboriginal and Torres Strait islander males – Implications for policy and practice. *American Journal of Men's Health., 14*, 155798832093612. https://doi.org/10.1177/1557988320936121

Statistics New Zealand. (2018). https://www.stats.govt.nz/tools/2018-census-ethnic-group-summaries/niuean

The National Hauora Coalition, Anderson, A., Brown, R., Wheeler, J., & Jansen, R. (2020). Pacific Fono: A community-based initiative to improve rheumatic fever service delivery for Pacific peoples in South Auckland. *Journal of Primary Health Care, 12*(4), 384–390.

Thomas, R. D. (2006). A general inductive approach for analyzing qualitative evaluation data. *American Journal of Evaluation, 27*, 237–246.

Chapter 13
"Been Through It Too": Exploring Community Development Through Collaborative Hip-Hop Creation

Roderick Wallace

Introduction

First of all, I am the youngest here to be honest wit' you… and I never really seen that none of my life… I can't really explain how to be a man... I ain't experience it myself, or feel the type of love from a man, you feel me? So, I would never in my life respect a man or a man trying to be my stepdaddy because I wouldn't want it at the end of the day because I never had my blood father to do it. You wanna know why? He said F me. So, it made me not respect no man on this Earth…I'm not saying every man not the same, but I just left it just like that.

Curious murmurs within the group of bearded Black faces rose into a fervor of daps, inquisitive looks, and affirming nods. We had been holding these discussion circles each week in the studio about topics that were close to the hearts of the men involved, but *this* was the one I had been waiting for. It was a crucible of sorts.

"There was a question … (that) his son asked him," responded a bespectacled man with a gruff voice. "'You didn't have a father… how did you turn out to be such a great father?' And the response was, 'I gave what I always wanted.' There are some things that you want from a man, some things from your father that you wanted... and now you are going to be in a position to say 'You know what? I'm going to do that.'"

The intergenerational dialogue above was from a community music project called Formula 734 (a reference to the local telephone area code), developed primarily by myself, a career educator and former high school principal, and Jamall Bufford, leader of Washtenaw County's (MI) branch of My Brother's Keeper from 2019–2020. This organization, also known as WMBK, is part of former President

R. Wallace (✉)
College of Education, Eastern Michigan University, Ypsilanti, MI, USA
e-mail: rwallac5@emich.edu

J. A. Smith et al. (eds.), *Health Promotion with Adolescent Boys and Young Men of Colour*, https://doi.org/10.1007/978-3-031-22174-3_13

Barack Obama's 2015 My Brother's Keeper initiative to "address persistent opportunity gaps facing boys and young men of colour and to ensure all youth can reach their full potential." WMBK's charge in brief was to advocate for the needs of young men of colour in Washtenaw County through mentorship, and intentional programming, and advocacy.

Both Jamall and I have a strong relationship with hip-hop as an artform, a culture, and a tool for critical expression. Jamall (or "Buff" as he was also known) had toured the world as a part of a hip-hop collective hip-hop artist for more than two decades, before working with students as a behaviour interventionist in the educational system. While teaching and leading schools in the metropolitan Detroit area for more than 20 years, I developed skills as a recording engineer and music producer as both a stress reliever and a dream. I also used hip-hop in my elementary and middle school classrooms throughout my career as a means of engaging students and a method of formative assessment.

After an opportunity to earn a doctorate in urban education presented itself, I chose to investigate the opportunities that hip-hop presents to the educational system to provide transferable skill development, creative liberation, and augmented agency for urban youth. After meeting Buff at a WMBK meeting in 2019, we discussed the possibilities of such a project grounded in hip-hop and collaboration to help the youth of the county experience career development in a different way. Buff eventually became the program specialist for WMBK, working with the county's educational authority and others to govern and lead the program. Soon after, we began crafting a project that would impact the lives and raise the voices of men in the area and embolden our resolve to be change agents in the community.

Hip-hop Song Writing and Beat Making as a Pathway to Agency

> "Life is a trip, and I'm out of this town,
>   The bottom of these J's have seen thousands of miles" – Michael (2020), 1:25.

A growing body of research involves hip-hop as praxis within the realms of social work, counselling, and personal development that acknowledges the positionality of hip-hop as a tool of engagement and a medium of self- expression for youth (Allen, p.30, 2005; Heath & Arroyo, 2014). Music therapy is not a new construct, as the nature of music has been used to speak to the inner cognitive and metacognitive processes for years, but a Eurocentric focus prevented access to other forms of music for this purpose (Elligan, 2004).

Hip-Hop Therapy (or HHT) is defined as a "culturally sensitive" method of engagement with youth that is a "synergy" of hip-hop music, music therapy, and narrative therapy (Tyson, 2002). To be clear, we were not administering therapy to the participants clinically or informally. However, engagement with the creative arts during group counselling strategies has demonstrated a reduction in stress (Martin et al., 2018), increasing insight and self-image (McCulliss & Chamberlain, 2013), and building community (Hermann-Turner et al., 2019). Our intent was grounded in the opportunity to engage the men in dialogue, providing them with a medium to express emotions and ideas in a format that could help them self-actualize their feelings.

Primarily, narrative therapy in a group setting would provide the backdrop for the creation of lyrical and conceptual content for F734. In narrative therapy, participants are encouraged to share their own viewpoints and stories regarding events, ideas, emotions, or themes. Heath and Arroyo (2014) believe that rap shares the floor as a "medium of expression" and can be used to tell "virtually any story." One of the key elements in engaging narrative therapy involving hip-hop is that those facilitating the experience and support must be well-versed in hip-hop and hip-hop culture (Heath & Arroyo, 2014). Both Buff and I have extensive experience and had an informal awareness of the cognitive engagement needed to stay on target in terms of content and meter, while also maintaining a connection with the listener and their experiences. Also, Saleeby (1993) points out the necessity of making it a "collaborative" experience; thus, we set basic terms and freely allow the participants to create.

Poetry also has value within this exercise because it gives creators opportunities to tap into hidden strengths. Poetry has a directly emotional relationship to self-empowerment, and can be used to describe and deconstruct oppression, taking on a different tonality and value (Furman et al., 2002). Our intent was to recognize introspective value to the listener but provide exponentially larger value to the writer and performer through the process of song writing ("rhyme writing" in hip-hop terms). The very nature of poetry is rhythmic, deeply introspective, and metaphorical. Wade (2000) posits that constructing poetry helps to free energy for personal development. Poetry has been a strengths-based approach in social work and other service-led fields and is part of a broader skill set known as bibliotherapy (Furman et al., 2002).

Like poetry, rhyme writing is metacognitive in that it expresses the writer's ideas and acquaints them with their thoughts simultaneously (Lerner, 1981). One key consideration for F734 is that because of the literal and direct nature of hip-hop music, it encourages the listener to deconstruct their own experiences through the words they hear. When the writer approaches the page, they are required to confront their truths about the topic and their feelings about those truths; they must also confront the rationale of each word in singularity and the necessity to be truthful, hyperbolic, or untruthful. Travis Jr et al. (2021) believes that hip-hop related creation, including song writing and beat making, allow for opportunities for catharsis and self-expression.

Ian Levy and Travis (2020) expands earlier concepts of Hip-Hop Therapy towards a theory of Hip-Hop Spoken Word Therapy (HHSWT) and provides a strong foundational framework through the lens of school counselling that can inform these excursions. Levy views the work of school counsellors in much the same manner that WMBK participants are encouraged to see themselves: as navigators, beacons of support, and drivers of individual and community growth. Levy created a system where students created lyric-based journals to process difficult thoughts or emotions, sharing them with the counsellor during the session. The counsellor then sought patterns of cognition and concomitant emotions to explore, offering feedback and suggestions to ensure that the author's words accurately reflected the ideas of the student. Levy also leverages collaborative work as a strategy, encouraging students to construct songs together on a common topic. This creates a space for emotional and intellectual safety among peers and encourages a shared approach to new meaning-making.

The resulting songs can be compiled into mixtapes, which are an important segment of hip-hop culture (Levy & Travis, 2020). Hip-hop mixtapes arose from the development of cassette technology early in the days of hip-hop, and to appear on a a prominent DJ or personality's tape was a badge of honour. These tapes were an amalgamation of audio clips, songs, freestyles (impromptu rap performances over random beats) and rap acapella recordings blended with different beats. The content is driven by common themes, ideas, or causes, and encompasses multiple perspectives on similar challenges, and new opportunities for artists and producers to collaborate. The essence of the mixtape ethos is captured through the last song on the F734 project, "Take Control," which is actually a remix from another project I was involved in called "East Grand," which has a reworked beat and some DJ scratches from Dr. Patrick McKay of Temple University.

Also key in this equation is hip-hop's ability to empower. Empowerment relates directly to an important element of hip-hop, which is knowledge of self (Akom, 2009). Constructivist approaches within hip-hop creation opportunities provide tiers of empowerment, including esteem, resilience, growth, community, and change (Travis Jr et al., 2021). By employing these elements in a hip-hop production experience for the men of F734, the benefits are twofold in that they gain insight into their own behaviours and develop solutions while also developing skills that transfer across different vocational and experiential planes. Travis et al. (2016) also says that this type of engagement qualifies as a self-care praxis for creators and promotes "health development."

Hip-hop: The Problem and the Solution

I got brothers on my side,
   I got brothers who ride,
   I got brothers who died,
   Gotta do what's right,
   Ain't just doing this for me,
   Doing this for me and my family,
   Niggas doing this for clout,
   And you had a lot of doubt,
   Guess what? I win,
   You could tell by the way that I grin,
   Can't do no gangs,
   That will have me in the grave.

Now thank the people.
That gave me the opportunity,
They gave me the way,
The way that they paved – Cooper (2020), 1:45.

We first must identify several distinctions particular to hip-hop when it is discussed in the realm of academic study, cultural critique, and practice. Hip-hop is a network of paradigms, responses, and concepts, bearing an important place within the realm of cultural production and critical discourse in America, particularly for people of colour. Hip-hop is a set of perspectives grounded in cultural ownership, self-expression, and independence (Akom, 2009). In the 19th and 20th centuries alone, Black Americans endured slavery, political persecution, wilful economic hegemony, an ethnocentric educational system, and outright attempts at genocide. Music has offered African-Americans opportunity for discourse, liberation, storytelling and hope for the entire thread of American history. Hip-hop arose as an emotional response from the young Black American man to the stressors of racism and poverty, in effect establishing "the Blackest culture" (Chang, 2005; Gilroy, 1997). Hip-hop subculture is mostly entered from the music created by the culture, which is the most-consumed music on the planet (Nzinga, 2018). A focus on its commercial merits, however, undermines other elements of hip-hop expression and cultural currency involved in hip-hop, and allows for its dominant narrative to be guided by its harshest criticisms first (Akom, 2009). The amoebic nature of culture in the time of mass media and globalism has spread hip-hop across the globe, and the music and culture has taken on the forms of where it rests primarily because of its "democratizing creative and aesthetic ethos" (Morgan & Bennett, 2011).

It is also clear that the didactic elements involved in hip-hop music provide an authentic opportunity for engaging with Black voices and interpretations as Black Americans are considered the key progenitors and drivers of the culture (Akom, 2009). Throughout the last quarter of the 1900s, hip-hop music gave specific insight and solution-based inquiry into the nuances of post-Civil Rights era/post-industrial Black America, where inner cities were plagued with drugs, crime, and poverty. During the 1980s, hip-hop music became a linchpin of Black critical discourse and meaning-making with seminal work by artists such as Grandmaster Melle Mel, Run DMC, and Boogie Down Productions providing sharp critique of social conditions (Hayman, 2013). As it gained the attention of middle-class White youth and the marketplace at-large, the profitability of the more controversial styles of hip-hop pushed fringe styles of the genre into the limelight, especially those that reinforced White stereotypes of Blacks (Kitwana, 2005). Songs and imagery that involved criminality, misogyny, and materialism would come to dominate the charts and the market-facing narrative about rap music during the 1990s, while more nuanced elements of the art form struggled to maintain market share (Akom, 2009). While mass media criticized hip-hop's content as maladaptive and as justification for oppressive and militaristic legislation, non-Black record labels, distributors, and publishing companies increasingly bound their fortune-seeking creators into predatory agreements – a sinister image of how White supremacy's exploitive complexity is braided into American capitalism (Karp, 2012).

However, the richness of the creative and iterative process of making hip-hop cannot be understated. Morgan and Bennett (2011) note that hip-hop brazenly encourages innovative expression of art, the production of knowledge, and social mobilisation as a movement for change. I regarded rappers as my heroes growing up as a young man interested in Afrocentrism and intellectual development. Through rap, I was introduced to Marcus Garvey, H. Rap Brown, and Louis Farrakhan.

I recognized early in my teaching career that my fluency in hip-hop gave me a means of access to my students and parents in a way that at the time was difficult to categorize. I was the DJ for many of the middle school parties, playing J Dilla instrumentals quietly in the background while students worked independently, and building programs that allowed students to engage with people from the music community. I even helped develop a full-fledged music production course that gave 125 students daily opportunities to make music and build important skills like marketing, collaboration, and user interface navigation. I viewed the students who rapped in my schools as some of the most brilliant people I had ever met; many, however, did not connect with the systemic approaches to school I was mandated to employ. As I gained traction as an educator and administrator grounded in culturally relevant practices, curriculum and content became more malleable first to me and then to those whom I would lead by my influence. These practices, as well as the literacies and social capital I juggled as a producer/engineer in the area's "rap scene," granted me a level of respect and access among my students and families. It was also an acknowledgment of my ability to exist in multiple spaces educationally without forsaking my professional reputation as an educational program developer, or my credibility as a listening ear and an advocate for non-traditional school achievement among the students I worked with.

After my transition into higher education, I sought scholarly opportunities to expand hip-hop as a kind of literacy, and to mine it for leadership and curricular constructs that could work in Black schools. This is how my generation told their stories, and I wanted the authentic voices of the young men of Washtenaw County to be heard. Giroux (2005) wrote that pedagogy "should focus on the creation of a public sphere" with the capacity to bring people together. I don't believe there is a better way than to use hip-hop for Black men, as it has now surpassed five decades of influence on our communities, yet it remains grounded in the movement of youth movements and culture (Pough, 2004). Urban education has recently emphasised more "culturally relevant" perspectives, practices, and pedagogy. In constructing cross-sector relationships with the private sector and governmental agencies to support low-income families, I have seen a similar emphasis on energizing ventures to support the needs of the community by engaging in the literacies of the community and empowering those in it to identify their needs. Therefore, the existing theoretical methodologies, praxes and other schools of thought informally embedded in F734 could potentially impact cross-sector community engagement and the lives of artists in our area via the long-term value of the project.

WMBK Formula 734

"Exceed what I believe that I could achieve/ I got dreams and I believe that I could succeed" – Greggs (2020), 1:25.

Washtenaw County, Michigan, sits at the nexus of racial and socioeconomic inequality. While African-Americans constitute 12% of the population of the county, and the county's overall poverty rate is 14%, African-Americans represent 19% of county residents living in poverty. Although Washtenaw County ranks the highest in Michigan of all counties in terms of access to health care (mostly because of Ann Arbor's University of Michigan, the state's largest employer) and is second in median household income, the life expectancy of its Black citizens is 13 years less than for its White citizens. In the cities of Ypsilanti and Ypsilanti Township, where much of WMBK's activity occurs, the discrepancy is 18 years between the eastern, mostly-Black region and the western, mostly White region (Robinson, 2021) of the county. While 93% of Ann Arbor residents have at least an associate's degree, only 13% of Ypsilanti's adults have achieved a similar distinction.

WMBK is a multi-faceted organization that specializes in grassroots community connectivity and social advocacy for issues surrounding men of colour. It is principally governed by a program specialist, a small planning committee, and a larger steering committee. These organizational bodies, composed of men of colour in the community, are engaged in some of the most powerful governmental and educational entities in the area. They are committed, however, to upholding the goals of the program. These goals include transforming communities of colour through growth and engagement, adjusting the perception and intra- and inter-ethnic narratives of men of colour, and creating financially sustainable spaces that eliminate barriers to success. Each month, the organization holds a "connecting breakfast" that includes dialogue, activities for children, and food at a community location. The organization has also extended its focus to create weekend leadership academies for children living in low-income housing, develop partnerships with other organizations of colour, and provide counsel and advocacy for public entities looking to engage with communities of colour on matters of equity.

Formula 734, or F734, was originally funded in 2018 as a media project to accurately depict the needs of men of colour in Washtenaw County and how WMBK meets those needs. The documentary that was created captured the ideas of young men in the area through interviews and artful editing. The interviewees discussed their aspirations, challenges, and dreams against a landscape of educational failure, disparate resources, and disconnected public systems.

When clips from the original project were shown at an event soon after its creation, Buff and I believed that there was an opportunity for a broader vision. What did the young men involved extract from the experience? How did that instance of engagement connect them closer to the program goals and tenets of not only WMBK, but within its community? Was there an opportunity to create something that could build upon itself, democratizing its own leadership and building a presence within the community that offered pathways of career readiness and self-reflection?

Buff and I decided to apply our combined energies to this project, engaging with local musicians and encouraging them to be thoughtful artists and reflexive community leaders simultaneously. We wanted to document their ideas and performances in a music album and capture the process in an accompanying documentary. Fred Culpepper of Creative Fluidity Productions was brought in to helm the video aspect of the project while WMBK planning committee member and entrepreneur Michael Henry came in as a producer and project manager. I volunteered to act as executive producer of the music album, while Buff administered the project overall. A local recording studio I directed and developed educational programs for partnered with WMBK to provide a space for the men to talk, have fellowship, and create music.

A few key ideas guided our team towards what we thought could be possible. First, we wanted to hear the unfettered, unedited voices of the young men. In identifying intellectual topics to tackle with them, we knew that their resulting words could create discomfort within certain power structures that were friendly with the organization. Our key supporters included county law enforcement, predominantly White institutions of higher education, the philanthropic community, and both the county's educational authority and governing commission. We made it clear from the beginning that the truth that they would bring was necessary and valued and would potentially only be edited for profanity. Second, the artists would have to be paid for their participation; this undid some of the perception that community art exists in a vacuum of limited resources, and indicated to the participants how serious their engagement was to us. We knew that the commitment of the men to our cause would be augmented by them seeing their value. Lastly, we entered the process with the intent of developing leadership amongst the ranks, pushing the young men to lead the project while we strategically moved into the background. This would develop them as leaders and voices within the community, ensuring that the project would continue to engage with new voices and new opportunities for years to come.

This project began very early on in my research journey, so I planned to apply some of the basic tenets of what I was being exposed to with what I knew as being best practices in the educational sector. This was not a study or an IRB-approved venture; rather, I was curious about the role of the academic in impacting the practice by attempting to apply a few theoretical frameworks and research nuggets to community projects. I was no stranger to leading collaborative music projects, but here was an opportunity to do so with a community focus and with my newfound presence as a hip-hop grounded educator in the hopes that such an opportunity could eventually lead to a possible dissertation topic.

I have always been interested in the production, recording, and development of popular music albums. I read record liner notes incessantly as a child, memorizing the individuals who assisted in making the album behind the scenes. That curiosity carried me into developing my skill set as a producer and an engineer, and from that perspective I could see the relationships, pitfalls, and victories involved in turning a fluid thought into an album.

With that in mind, I sought to answer a few key questions. How is hip-hop used as a source of critical discourse and meaning-making among youth, primarily Black men? How can the creation of hip-hop music (used interchangeably with rap music), and more so the creation of a compiled hip-hop album or project, be used as a platform for collaborating, developing transferable skills, and engaging young men in the community? Lastly, what are the implications for mental health and educational practitioners looking for innovative methods to engage with young Black men and construct a space of emotional and intellectual safety towards individual and collective goals involving self-awareness and enhanced emotional control?

Setting the Stage

As the idea came to fruition, Buff and I began thinking through potential candidates for participation. Each person who was invited to participate had some sort of connection to me or Buff. He had several candidates from his engagement with similar music-focused programs in the area in the past. Each participant had to commit to at least 8 bimonthly meetings and participation in WMBK meetings in order to be paid.

The participants ranged in age from 16 to 52 and came from very diverse backgrounds. Many of the participants also brought distinct skill sets to the table for the project, with expertise in photography, audio engineering and production, and music theory. Our intent was to capture the richness and full measure of their skills to create an album while also illustrating how these skill sets can be used in other areas to augment their career aspirations or entrepreneurial opportunities.

Each session began with sharing food and soft drinks with the participants, during which any updates on the project could be shared or simple well-wishes could be exchanged. The studio, a repurposed industrial office space, had several rooms that could be used for different purposes. Some spaces were specifically used for production and recording, while other spaces allowed the videographer to do one-on-one interviews of participants.

Each session began with a reminder and an assessment of our group norms. The norms included "One mic," meaning that only one person could speak at a time; and "No hating," which both acknowledged the participants' allegiances outside of the venture as well as the importance of maintaining a positive and emotionally transparent atmosphere.

As each session began, the participants and guests were welcomed to sit in a circle. Buff and I both believed that discussion circles would need to be an important part of this program. When I was introduced to them several years ago as a high school administrator, such circles helped curb out-of-school suspensions by almost 30%. Buff had been trained to facilitate restorative circles with students in conflict as a behaviour interventionist. As we approached the start of the program, I did some broader research regarding healing circles. Within the context of Indigenous North American peoples, discussion circles were designed and governed to prevent interruptions and to ensure that every voice was heard. Among the Lakota nation, these group circles are referred to as "hocokah," according to Mehl-Madrona and Mainguy (2014), a process that stimulates "multicultural awareness while fostering respect for individual differences and facilitating group cohesion."

The conversations were typically led by open-ended questions such as, "How would you change if you were to be successful?" or "When you consider the image of a man, what do you see? Who set the example for you?" A pad and marker were used to capture main themes extracted from the conversation. As the discussions commenced, we asked the artists follow-up questions that allowed them the opportunity to expound and dig deeper into their own experiences in a reflective manner.

We did not look to control the process to the degree that it could potentially stifle the process or the outcomes. However, there are several elements from this experience that align with frameworks supporting different areas of self-expression and self-reflection. Allen (2005) also outlines a "person-in-environment" approach that engages the participants in seeing their experiences within the broader contexts of where and how they occurred. The facilitator placed the locus of control firmly in the hands of the participants.

After recording the music, I would be charged with moulding the songs, audio clips, and instrumentation into a cohesive, 45-minute audio experience. This process occurred during the COVID-19 crisis of 2020, though most of the audio had been compiled before the pandemic. After mixing and mastering the album, the album was uploaded to streaming sites on July 31, 2020 (Fig. 13.1).

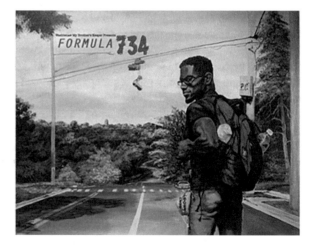

Fig. 13.1 Formula 734 Cover. Painting by Curtis Wallace, @cwcreatyv

Outcomes

> Transparency is talked about but rarely seen,
>   Walk the walk from Pine Lake to Danbury Green,
>   734, call it Ypsi Deuce,
>   20 years, been in my bag like Big League Chew – Bufford (2020), Track 12, 1:40.

Pine Lake Cooperative Apartments, a housing project with a high percentage of impoverished Black residents, can be found on the northern edge of Ann Arbor in an area that is relatively affluent. Danbury Green, seemingly on the opposite side of Washtenaw County proper in eastern Ypsilanti, has the same characteristics. The above passage, performed by program specialist Bufford himself on the song "Take Control," highlights the pervasiveness of poverty and how it can even be found in one of the richest areas of the state. Ypsilanti and Ann Arbor are typically viewed as two separate entities because of the perceived division in their histories and labels. This illustrates how issues of income inequality are much more far-reaching than many understand, and how the cities' destinies are aligned.

This highlighted one of the biggest takeaways from this project. Hip-hop is affixed to places just as music is affixed to time. I noticed how we subconsciously grounded this work in the place where it was created. From the sounds of trains going by in the middle of songs to the sounds of men laughing in a barbershop during an interlude, we were able to capture the young men's ideas as well as the time and place. The collaborative album process – or "mixtape," if you will – connects the community to the art it fosters in a very unique and authentic way.

The album was recorded between November 2019 and March 2020, when in-person sessions were abruptly cut short by the COVID-19 pandemic. Although the pandemic limited our face-to-face engagement, we still found a way to release the album during the summer of 2020 as originally planned on July 31, 2020. It is currently available on all streaming platforms as well as formula734.com. The accompanying documentary has made the rounds of a few film festivals and has been shown multiple times within Washtenaw County in the hope of finding an opportunity for a broader release.

Over the five months that we recorded, many participants described the experience as transformative. The artists, instrumentalists, producers, and engineers developed a kinship rooted in community and ownership of community. The artists developed working relationships beyond the walls of the studio, and the producers and mentors of the venture were able to expose the brilliance of the young men involved to the broader community in the area.

There is a strong grounding for further qualitative study regarding collaborative music creation as community building work for organizations. As executive producer and the "resident academic," this pilot program exhibited a lot of room to grow and frame further research.

By relying on song writing and the creation of hip-hop as a strength-based and reflexive practice of young Black men, our hope was to provide the men with a mirror to show them who they are and who they hope to be. What we found was an even more definitive pathway towards informing community organizations and agencies about how to communicate, engage, and leverage the strengths of Black men in community development. The content of the conversations reframes widely held narratives about Black men in Washtenaw County and elsewhere. In reviewing the very pointed conversations that occurred before recording, we saw that the intimate setup, positive yet politely competitive environment, discussion norms, and intentional cultural development paid off in a level of honesty and vulnerability that made the project special. Using the experience and the resulting album and documentary, we began to engage with local universities, county organizations, and schools about the experience and what it tells us about communicating effectively with men from the neighbourhoods.

Secondly, we must highlight the importance of proper facilitation. The relationships established by Buff and the other adults, and the cultural capital we brought to the young men as hip-hop-fluent adults and authority figures, opened up the experience for the young men. It is essential that facilitators demonstrate literacy in hip-hop as well as an interest in developing the participants individually and collectively. The participants must see that the facilitators understand the broader context of what they intend to create, but are centred in accelerating participants' development.

Lastly, future studies of this work would benefit from the involvement of mental health professionals as participants in the discussions; added support mechanisms for artists who want to utilize this opportunity to purge emotions and ideas; and informing and assessing the process along the way. By embedding strategies from narrative and poetry therapy, as well as Hip-hop Spoken Word Therapy, we can engage participants in a life-changing activity that gives the men of our area voice and provides the community with hope.

References

Akom, A. A. (2009). Critical hip-hop pedagogy as a form of liberatory praxis. *Equity & Excellence in Education, 42*(1), 52–66.

Allen, N. M. T. (2005). Exploring hip-hop therapy with high-risk youth. *Building on Our Foundations, 5*(1), 30–36.

Bufford, J. (2020). Take control. In *On Formula 734*. Project Plugin.

Chang, J. (2005). *Can't stop, won't stop: A history of the hip-hop generation*. St. Martin's Press.

Cooper, D. (2020). Pavement. In *On Formula 734*. Project Plugin.

Elligan, D. (2004). *Rap therapy: A practical guide for communicating with youth and young adults through rap music*. Kensington Publishing Corporation.

Furman, R., Downey, E. P., Jackson, R. L., & Bender, K. (2002). Poetry therapy as a tool for strengths-based practice. *Advances in Social Work, 3*(2), 146–157.

Gilroy, P. (1997). "After the love has gone": Bio-politics and etho-poetics in the black public sphere. In A. McRobbie (Ed.), *Back to reality? Social experience and cultural studies* (pp. 83–115). Manchester University Press.

Giroux, H. (2005). *Border crossings: Cultural workers and the politics of education*. Routledge.

Greggs, T. J. (2020). Grown. In *On Formula 734*. Project Plugin.

Hayman, C. (2013). Melle Mel in the Megaplex: Postmodern performance and the hip-hop "real" in" Krush groove" &" beat street.". *African American Review, 46*(1), 117–132.

Heath, T., & Arroyo, P. (2014). 'I gracefully grab a pen and embrace it': Hip-hop lyrics as a means for re-authoring and therapeutic change. *International Journal of Narrative Therapy & Community Work, 3*, 31–38.

Hermann-Turner, K. M., Heyward, K. J., & Bailey, C. L. (2019). Community uprising: Counseling interventions, educational strategies, and advocacy tools. *The Journal of Counselor Preparation and Supervision, 12*(1), 1–19.

Karp, J. (2012). 6. Blacks, Jews, and the business of race music, 1945-1955. In R. Kobrin (Ed.), *Chosen Capital* (pp. 141–167). Rutgers University Press.

Kitwana, B. (2005). *Why white kids love hip-hop: Wankstas, wiggers, wannabes, and the new reality of race in America*. Civitas Books.

Lerner, A. (1981). Poetry therapy. In R. Corsini (Ed.), *Handbook of innovative psychotherapies* (pp. 131–152). John Wiley.

Levy, I., & Travis, R. (2020). The critical cycle of mixtape creation: Reducing stress via three different group counseling styles. *The Journal for Specialists in Group Work, 45*(4), 307–330.

Martin, L., Oepen, R., Bauer, K., Nottensteiner, A., Mergheim, K., Gruber, H., & Koch, S. (2018). Creative arts interventions for stress management and prevention—A systematic review. *Behavioral Sciences, 8*(2), 28. https://doi.org/10.3390/bs8020028

McCulliss, D., & Chamberlain, D. (2013). Bibliotherapy for youth and adolescents—School-based application and research. *Journal of Poetry Therapy, 26*(1), 13–40.

Mehl-Madrona, L., & Mainguy, B. (2014). Introducing healing circles and talking circles into primary care. *The Permanente Journal, 18*(2), 4–9.

Michael, T. (2020). Be like this. In *On Formula 734*. Project Plugin.

Morgan, M., & Bennett, D. (2011). Hip-hop & the global imprint of a black cultural form. *Daedalus, 140*(2), 176–196.

Nzinga, K. L. K. (2018). The social conscience of rap: What young people learn from hip-hop about everyday ethics. *Available from ProQuest Dissertations & Theses Global*, 2267452576.

Pough, G. D. (2004). *Check it while I wreck it: Black woman-hood, hip-hop culture, and the public sphere*. Northeastern University Press.

Robinson, S. (2021). "Opportunity Index 'first step' in addressing inequities across Washtenaw County, leaders say." https://www.mlive.com/news/ann-arbor/2021/05/opportunity-index-first-step-in-addressing-inequities-across-washtenaw-county-leaders-say.html

Saleeby, D. (1993). *The strengths perspective in social work practice*.

Travis, R., Bowman, S. W., Childs, J., & Villanueva, R. (2016). Musical interactions: Girls who like and use rap music for empowerment. In *Symbolic interactionist takes on music* (Vol. 47, pp. 119–149). Emerald Group Publishing Limited.

Travis, R., Jr., Gann, E., Crooke, A. H., & Jenkins, S. M. (2021). Using therapeutic beat making and lyrics for empowerment. *Journal of Social Work, 21*(3), 551–574.

Tyson, E. H. (2002). Hip-hop therapy: An exploratory study of a rap music intervention with at-risk and delinquent youth. *Journal of Poetry Therapy, 15*(3), 133–144.

Wade, R. C. (2000). Service-learning for multicultural teaching competency: Insights from the literature for teacher educators. *Equity & Excellence in Education, 33*(3), 21–29.

Chapter 14
Masculinities and Health in Justice-Involved Youth: Implications for Boys and Young Men of Colour

John Bosco, Christopher Bondoc, Elizabeth S. Barnert, and Jocelyn I. Meza

Introduction: Background

The United States (U.S.) juvenile justice population is well known to be disproportionately composed of Black and Latinx males from low-income communities. Compared to adult incarceration, juvenile incarceration is distinct in that it theoretically prioritizes rehabilitation before punishment. However, much controversy remains regarding whether and how correctional systems and their curricula achieve their goal of rehabilitation (Chambers & Balck, 2014; National Research Council, 2012). In its current state, juvenile incarceration unfortunately separates families, disrupts career and education trajectories, and substantially burdens marginalized communities of colour (Braverman & Morris, 2011; Dumont et al., 2012). Moreover, many authors have noted associations between justice involvement and serious health concerns, such as post-traumatic stress disorder (PTSD), death from suicide, and drug overdose (Binswanger et al., 2007; Haney, 2001). Justice involvement has also been linked to worse long-term health outcomes, including depression and

J. Bosco (✉)
Department of Pediatrics, David Geffen School of Medicine, University of California, Los Angeles, CA, USA

Department of Emergency Medicine, Harbour-UCLA Medical Center, Torrance, CA, USA
e-mail: jbosco@dhs.lacounty.gov

C. Bondoc · E. S. Barnert
Department of Internal Medicine & Pediatrics, David Geffen School of Medicine, University of California, Los Angeles, CA, USA
e-mail: cbondoc@mednet.ucla.edu; ebarnert@mednet.ucla.edu

J. I. Meza
Department of Psychiatry, University of California, Los Angeles, CA, USA
e-mail: JIMeza@mednet.ucla.edu

J. A. Smith et al. (eds.), *Health Promotion with Adolescent Boys and Young Men of Colour*, https://doi.org/10.1007/978-3-031-22174-3_14

functional limitations into adulthood (Barnert et al., 2017), as well as infectious diseases such as tuberculosis and HIV (Farmer, 2002; Massoglia & Remster, 2019). Further, these health disparities are often amplified by high rates of re-arrest and repeated incarceration among justice-involved youth, with scholars estimating the rate of re-arrest to be as a high as 45–75% (Greenwood, 1996; Lipsey, 2000; Snyder & Sickmund, 2006).

Incarceration and Health

Several factors contribute to the significant health burden faced by justice-involved youth during incarceration, community re-entry after incarceration, and throughout their life course post-incarceration. Notably, there is not a clear causal relationship between incarceration and health; many social determinants of health, such as poverty and specific health conditions (e.g., behavioural health disorders), are associated with an increased risk of incarceration (Barnert et al., 2016; Schnittker & John, 2007). However, there are still some widely accepted, plausible theories purporting a causal relationship between incarceration and health. To start, some authors have described incarceration itself as a traumatic experience (Akyüz et al., 2007; Vaswani et al., 2021; Welfare & Hollin, 2015), as it leads to feelings of stigmatization, alienation from society, and hopelessness. Others have described how justice-involved youth often have histories of untreated trauma, which might then impede their ability to cope with the additional trauma of incarceration (Van Der Kolk, 2014). As such, incarceration itself likely exacerbates or even causes serious health burden for youth who already marginalized and tasked with overcoming numerous barriers to their health and re-entry success.

Healthcare and Community Re-entry After Incarceration

Some authors have emphasised that youth undergoing community re-entry after incarceration face the "dual transition" of reintegrating into society while simultaneously transitioning from adolescence to adulthood (Altschuler & Brash, 2004). Despite the juvenile justice system's supposed intent to rehabilitate, current programming often leaves youth ill-prepared to deal with the challenges awaiting them once they leave incarceration (Nurse et al., 2018) – allowing existing health concerns to worsen and impede re-entry success. However, providing healthcare during the six-month re-entry window has been found to reduce recidivism, improve both educational and vocational outcomes (Bullis et al., 2004; Chung et al., 2007) and promote mental and physical wellbeing (Wang et al., 2012). Still, substantial gaps in treatment exist during the critical re-entry period, particularly with behavioural and reproductive health (Binswanger et al., 2007; Montague et al., 2012; Rich et al., 2011). In addition to gaps in care continuity and low service uptake, some studies have shown that juvenile justice youth drop out of post-incarceration programming and support more than adults (Needels et al., 2004). Even when youth do connect with care, ensuring they continue to receive support and engage with treatment presents challenges.

Addressing Healthcare Needs

There are several steps that can be taken to alleviate the health burden of incarceration. To start, it is critical to understand how carceral environments could better address the needs of justice-involved youth, particularly for behavioural health challenges such substance use and trauma. It is also crucial that justice-involved youth receive adequate support in connecting with healthcare post-incarceration and engaging in health-promoting behavioural changes such as reduced substance use, safe sex practices, medication compliance, and improved diet and exercise. Given that the vast majority of incarcerated youth identify as male, it follows that gender identity might play an important role in program design. Many of the healthcare challenges that disproportionately affect justice-involved males are also more prevalent among men more generally, namely substance use, death from suicide, HIV, and heart disease (Heilman et al., 2017; Ragonese et al., 2019). However, gender-sensitive programs are rarely delivered in correctional settings (Abrams et al., 2008; Vaswani et al., 2021). Despite their unique healthcare needs, males of all ages more commonly delay help-seeking, forego treatment altogether, and fail to obtain a regular source of healthcare (Addis & Mahalik, 2003; Cherry et al., 2007; Mansfield et al., 2003; Sandman et al., 2000). Thus, there is clear need to develop more gender-sensitive approaches to rehabilitation in correctional settings.

Masculinities and Men of Colour

A gender-sensitive approach to rehabilitation amongst justice-involved youth would require applying current research on the gender-based attitudes and behaviours of justice involved young men. These gender-based attitudes and behaviours are often referred to as Masculinities. Masculinities are defined as attitudes and behaviours commonly endorsed by men as contributing to their sense of gender identity, and this framework can be used to help understand masculinity and health. First, a brief review of the masculinity discourse is helpful to understand how a masculinities framework might help promote health, especially since the research tools traditionally used to study masculinities have more recently drawn criticism. In the 1970s, researchers began to identify behavioural and psychological themes common to men, with the underlying assumption that sex assigned at birth played a major role in health behaviours (Smiler, 2004). Much of the initial research focused on identifying attitudes commonly endorsed by men, sometimes referred to as masculine norms, with more recent studies looking at the impact these attitudes have on men's health-related behaviours (Broom & Tovey, 2009; Robertson, 2007). However, most research has shown that men's adherence to masculine norms produces mixed effects; sometimes endorsement of masculine norms is health protective, while at other times it detracts from health (Griffith et al., 2012). Researchers also now acknowledge that the masculinities discourse generally has a negativity bias (i.e., an under-examination of health-related attitudes that may be health-protective). There are continued efforts to expand the understanding of how masculine norms operate in different contexts, such as in carceral settings (Daniels et al., 2009) and among marginalized and minoritized groups, including specific races, ethnicities, and sexual orientations (Griffith et al., 2012; Nurse et al., 2018). Thus, current limitations of the literature, including a lack of intersectional approaches and general negativity bias in existing scales and tools, restrict the value of masculine norms as a lens to improve the health of incarcerated males.

In response to limitations in the extant literature, more recent work has focused on masculinities among men of colour to expand intersectional understanding of how masculine norms operate in various groups and communities (Griffith et al., 2012). A 2012 review by Griffith and colleagues examined which masculine norm scales had been utilized to study men of colour, with the majority of the reviewed scales commonly being used across a broad range races and ethnicities. They found that the most commonly-utilized scales included: Male Role Norms Inventory, Conformity to Masculine Norms Inventory, and Male Gender Role Stress. Notably, scale use varied greatly between health outcomes. In general, they found that greater endorsement of masculine attitudes was positively associated with drug use, depressive symptoms, alexithymia, stress, and reduced help-seeking behaviours (Griffith et al., 2012). Machismo was also a commonly used framework, and was one of the few examples of masculine norms scales used to describe a specific ethnicity. Machismo, a subtype of masculinity identified among Mexican men, is described as including hyper-masculine traits, like dominance, in addition to nurturing qualities such as family-centeredness (Arciniega et al., 2008). Arciniega et al. (2008) articulated a distinction between traditional Machismo and Caballerismo, with Caballerismo focusing more on emotional connection with family members. Numerous qualitative studies have also explored the definitions of manhood amongst Black men. A 2020 study exploring racial and gender identity among Black male youth showed that many young Black men defined their manhood through personal responsibility and emotional expression, with several endorsing emotional restriction as a sign of manhood (Quam et al., 2020). However, other studies have shown that compassion, humanism, and authenticity are crucial to gender identity among Black men (Ford, 2011). Taken together, these studies highlight the variability of masculinities amongst different groups, the fluid and sometimes paradoxical definitions of masculine norms, and the challenge of developing general scales and theoretical frameworks to understand how masculine norms operate to influence health and wellbeing.

Vignette 14.1: Interview with Black and Latinx Male Youth

The following vignette was generated based on real interviews conducted with Black and Latinx male youth undergoing re-entry after incarceration in Los Angeles, California. Dialogue represents common features of interviews with male youth, which researchers believed emphasised the role played by masculine norms in the lives of juvenile male youth exiting the juvenile justice system.

Vignette:

Therapist: So, how have things been since we last met?

Sam: Things have been cool.

Therapist: Things have been cool?

Sam: Yeah, you know, just more of the same. Same old stuff.

Therapist: And what's the "same old stuff"?

Sam: Just, you know—Wake up, do my thing, repeat.

Therapist: Ok, so would you say things are going well then?

Sam: I mean, things aren't like great. It's not like things are perfect. But, at the same time, nothing terrible is going on, you know? Feel like I can't complain.

Therapist: I hear that, and I'm glad to hear nothing terrible is happening. But, in terms of things being "not great," do you want to tell me more about that?

Sam: Not really, if I'm being honest.

Therapist: That's fair, and I appreciate your honesty. Do you mind if ask why not?

Sam: It's just like… I don't like talking about that kind of stuff.

Therapist: And what's "that kind of stuff"?

Sam: Like how I'm feeling. I don't really get into all that. I mean, they made me talk to someone in juvenile hall and it was cool, I guess… but still weird. I mean maybe it helped but—I don't know. I'm just not used to it, I guess. Like, I barely know this person. Why am I going to tell them my whole life story?

Therapist: I can understand that. Well, how about we check-in on some of those goals we had set at our last session?

Sam: I'm not going to lie, I totally forgot about them.

Therapist: That's ok, I think it'll still be good to check in. How about you remind me what those goals were and what you think maybe got in the way of you remembering them?

Sam: I think we talked about me trying new ways to relax instead of smoking because I don't want to get in trouble with probation for a dirty test or anything like that.

Therapist: Mhm.

Sam: Yeah… I don't know what happened, really. I just kind of felt like doing it to be honest, I guess I was just stressed. It's hard to do something new when I have to do all these things—See the judge at court, check in with probation, figure out how to get started at a new school. It's a bunch of things. And then make me go to all these appointments on top of all that, no offense.

Therapist: None taken. That sounds like a lot of work. Do you have anyone who helps you with all of that?

Sam: Not really. Like, I'm not a kid anymore, I'm a man, I have to be able to figure things out on my own. So, I don't know. I feel like it's just on me. Well… sometimes, my girlfriend will ask me how things are going now that I'm back or if she can help with some of my stuff that I got going on. I don't even have to tell her like "hey, I need help" or anything weird like that. And I don't feel like bothering my parents.

Therapist: That's great that she helps you so much. What about your friends, are they able to help you out sometimes as well?

Sam: I don't know. It's just like, us guys, you know? Because this is more like, "I'm feeling stressed" or "I'm worried about this or that," and I don't talk to them about that kind of stuff.

Note the emotional restriction the patient shows, often describing his feelings as neutral initially, and later acknowledging negative feelings after some focused questioning. In addition, note Sam's lack of concern about his marijuana use, despite risks to his probation, as well as his minimal social support.

Masculinities and Justice Involvement

There is limited research on masculinities and health among justice-involved youth, with the existing literature focusing primarily on how incarceration can reinforce masculine norms relating to worse health outcomes. This research often focuses on the reinforcement of hegemonic masculinities specifically, which refers to behaviours and attitudes generally considered to be dominant or ideal in a particular culture at a particular time (Connell, 1995). Evidence from qualitative research suggests that detention and incarceration reinforce health-detracting masculine norms through the structure of their physical environments, daily activities, and interactions with guards.

Physical Environment

In regard to physical environments, distance from families and the structural characteristics of detention facilities play important roles in reinforcing particular masculine norms. Several researchers have observed how separation from families during incarceration might reinforce health-detracting masculinities by limiting youth exposure to positive role modelling from family members (Abrams et al., 2008; Cox, 2011; Fader, 2013). Many authors have also noted that specific structural elements such as bright lights, overcrowding, and constant noise can trigger symptoms of PTSD (Jewkes, 2011; Miller & Najavits, 2012). At the same time, some researchers have noted that men with histories of trauma frequently exert exaggerated displays of hegemonic masculine norms to reassert power and control (Elder et al., 2017; Ellis et al., 2017). Routine strip searches and daily threats of violence may have similar effects and result in increased aggression, violence, and risk-taking (Miller & Najavits, 2012).

Daily Activity

Daily activities in juvenile correctional facilities can also reinforce hegemonic masculinities. In many facilities, researchers have observed that daily activities typically consist of competitive sports or games. This focus on physical competition then reinforces social hierarchies predicated on physical size and toughness (Abrams et al., 2008; Nurse et al., 2018). As such, these researchers assert that juvenile correctional facilities lack adequate programs and activities where youth can engage in alternative forms of gendered expression, such as artistic development or academic advancement. Other researchers have noted alternative forms of gender identity among incarcerated youth, suggesting that different masculine norms can be encouraged to become widespread in any given correctional facility. For example, in a study examining masculine identity among Black and Latinx male youth, researchers found that participants viewed emotional expression as a strength, instead of emotional restriction (Quam et al., 2020). In an intervention involving open discussions with youth, researchers then leveraged this youth value to reduce substance use, HIV risk, and violence exposure, highlighting the potential of integrating similar programming in juvenile correctional facilities. Youth may benefit from opportunities and programming allowing for and/or leveraging alternative forms of gendered expression.

Correctional Staff Interactions

Correctional staff may reinforce health-detracting masculine norms. For example, correctional staff have been observed allowing the use of misogynistic and/or homophobic messages among male youth (Abrams et al., 2008; Vaswani et al., 2021). Researchers have also observed correctional staff modelling emotional restriction while simultaneously discouraging open emotional expression in youth. However, correctional staff can play a role in facilitating alternative, more health-promoting masculine norms as well. Some interventions for justice-involved youth have demonstrated value in encouraging correctional staff to role model emotional awareness and speak to their own identities (Daniels et al., 2009). Given the high prevalence of trauma in the juvenile justice population, such interventions might also help young men with histories of trauma learn to express themselves and ultimately encourage engagement in needed behavioural health treatment or support (Vaswani et al., 2021).

Some researchers have asserted that correctional facilities might benefit from disseminating and implementing gender-sensitive mental health interventions (Abrams et al., 2008; Quam et al., 2020; Ragonese et al., 2019). While justice-involved males are well known to have high rates of adverse child experiences (ACEs) and PTSD (Vaswani et al., 2021), males with PTSD generally show more limited engagement in treatment and worse treatment outcomes (Morrison, 2012; Shields, 2016; Wade et al., 2016). Some researchers have then argued that men may show worse engagement in behavioural health treatment because doing so directly contradicts certain hegemonic masculine norms (Elder et al., 2017; Mejia, 2005). Thus, programs that consider and address concerns related to masculine identity might improve treatment engagement among justice-involved males. Some scholars have suggested potential in leveraging masculine identity in behavioural health treatment to promote overall health. Current intervention mainly utilizes cognitive behavioural therapy (CBT), which aims to challenge and restructure thought associated with distressful symptoms and behaviours. While evidence-based interventions, such as CBT, have been effective in research settings, many advocates have noted that these treatments often disregard the numerous barriers to care faced by justice-involved youth, including structural barriers (e.g., systemic racism, poverty, and lack of access) and psychosocial barriers such as negative attitudes towards treatment (Abrams et al., 2008; Nurse et al., 2018). Given that hegemonic masculine attitudes directly contradict engagement in behavioural health treatment, future work might focus on considering and addressing masculine norms in order to promote the health and success of justice-involved male youth.

Conclusion

Justice-involved youth are at increased risk of both acute and chronic adverse health outcomes, including overdose, death from suicide, HIV, and more limited adult functioning. Prior to incarceration, these youth already disproportionately experience poverty, systemic racism, and trauma, which likely contribute to and worsen already concerning health disparities. Correctional facilities can potentially mitigate these health concerns through safer physical environments, improved programming, and gender-sensitive interventions. There is emerging literature on our intersectional understanding of masculinities in the context of different races, sexual orientations, and gender identities. Simultaneously, there is a need to improve research tools to better observe masculinities in various groups and communities. While there is mixed evidence on the effect of any single masculine norm, the majority of research signals that high adherence to composite masculine norms scales likely impedes health, through lowered healthcare utilization and delayed help-seeking. Though much of the existing literature points to the ways in which masculine norms detract health, research on the value of promoting alternative masculinities offers a promising pathway for harnessing youth identity to instead promote their long-term health and success. As such, continued research on masculinities and health among justice-involved youth might help to redress health disparities and other inequities in the population. Future efforts should focus on developing more gender-sensitive health interventions in justice-involved male youth, as well as expanding our understanding of how these young men define manhood.

References

Abrams, L. S., Anderson-Nathe, B., & Aguilar, J. (2008). Constructing masculinities in juvenile corrections. *Men and Masculinities, 11*(1), 22–41.

Addis, M. E., & Mahalik, J. R. (2003). Men, masculinity, and the contexts of help seeking. *American Psychologist, 58*(1), 5–14.

Akyüz, G., Kuğu, N., Şar, V., & Doğan, O. (2007). Trauma and dissociation among prisoners. *Nordic Journal of Psychiatry, 61*, 167–172.

Altschuler, D. M., & Brash, R. (2004). Adolescent and teenage offenders confronting the challenges and opportunities of re-entry. *Youth Violence and Juvenile Justice, 2*(1), 72–87.

Arciniega, G. M., Anderson, T. C., Tovar-Blank, Z. G., & Tracey, T. J. G. (2008). Toward a fuller conception of machismo: Development of a traditional machismo and caballerismo scale. *Journal of Counseling Psychology, 55*(1), 19–33.

Barnert, E. S., Perry, R., & Morris, R. E. (2016). Juvenile incarceration and health. *Academic Pediatrics., 16*(2), 99–109. pmid:26548359.

Barnert, E. S., et al. (2017). How does incarcerating young people affect their adult health outcomes? *Pediatrics, 139*(2), e20162624. https://doi.org/10.1542/peds.2016-2624. PMID: 28115536; PMCID: PMC5260153.

Binswanger, I. A., Stern, M. F., Deyo, R. A., et al. (2007). Release from prison--a high risk of death for former inmates. *New England Journal of Medicine, 356*(2), 157–165. pmid:17215533.

Braverman, P., & Morris, R. (2011). The health of youth in the juvenile justice system. In F. Sherman & F. Jacobs (Eds.), *Juvenile justice – Advancing research, policy, and practice* (pp. 44–67). Wiley.

Broom, A., & Tovey, P. (2009). Men's health: Body. In U. K. Chichester (Ed.), *Identity, & social context* (pp. 1–5). Wiley-Blackwell.

Bullis, M., Yovanoff, P., Mueller, G., & Havel, E. (2004). The importance of getting started right: Further examination of the facility-to-community transition of formerly incarcerated youth. *Journal of Special Education, 38*(2), 80–94.

Chambers, B., & Balck, A. (2014). *Because kids are different: Five opportunities for reforming the juvenile justice system*. Macarthur Foundation.

Cherry, D. K., Woodwell, D. A., & Rechtsteiner, E. A. (2007). National Ambulatory Medical Care Survey: 2005 summary. *Advance Data, 2007*(387), 1–39.

Chung, H. L., Schubert, C. A., & Mulvey, E. P. (2007). An empirical portrait of community re-entry among serious juvenile offenders in two metropolitan cities. *Criminal Justice and Behavior, 34*(11), 1402–1426.

Connell, R. W. (1995). *Masculinities*. Polity Press.

Cox, A. (2011). Doing the programme or doing me? The pains of youth imprisonment. *Punishment & Society, 13*(5), 592–610.

Daniels, J., et al. (2009). Creating real men: Description of an intervention to reduce drug use, HIV risk, and rearrest among young men returning to urban communities from jail. *Health Promotion Practice, 12*(1), 44–54.

Dumont, D. M., Brockmann, B., Dickman, S., et al. (2012). Public health and the epidemic of incarceration. *Annual Review of Public Health, 33*, 325–339.

Elder, W. B., Domino, J. L., Mata-Galán, E. L., et al. (2017). Masculinity as an avoidance symptom of posttraumatic stress. *Psychology of Men & Masculinity, 18*, 198–207.

Ellis, A., Winlow, S., & Hall, S. (2017). 'Throughout my life I've had people walk all over me': Trauma in the lives of violent men. *The Sociological Review, 65*, 699–713.

Fader, J. J. (2013). *Falling back: Incarceration and transitions to adulthood among urban youth*. Rutgers University Press.

Farmer, P. (2002). The house of the dead: Tuberculosis and incarceration. In M. Mauer & M. Chesney-Lind (Eds.), *Invisible punishment: The collateral consequences of mass imprisonment* (pp. 239–257). The New Press.

Ford, K. A. (2011). Doing fake masculinity, being real men: Present and future constructions of self among black college men. *Symbolic Interaction, 34*, 38–62.

Greenwood, P. (1996). Responding to juvenile crime: Lessons learned. *Future of Children, 6*(3), 75–85.

Griffith, D. M., Gunter, K., & Watkins, D. C. (2012). Measuring masculinity in research on men of colour: Findings and future directions. *American Journal of Public Health, 102*(Suppl. 2), S187–S194. https://doi.org/10.2105/AJPH.2012.300715

Haney, C. (2001). *The psychological impact of incarceration: Implications for post-prison adjustment*. U.S. Department of Health and Human Services.

Heilman, B., Barker, G., & Harrison, A. (2017). *The man box: A study on being a young man in the U.S., U.K., and Mexico*. Promundo-US and Unilever.

Jewkes, Y. (2011). Loss, liminality and the life sentence: Managing identity through a disrupted lifecourse. In A. Liebling & S. Maruna (Eds.), *The effects of imprisonment* (pp. 366–388). Routledge.

Lipsey, M. W. (2000). *What 500 intervention studies show about the effects of intervention on the recidivism of juvenile offenders.* Paper presented at the Annual Conference on Criminal Justice Research and Evaluation, Washington, D.C., July 16–19.

Mansfield, A. K., Addis, M. E., & Mahalik, J. R. (2003). "Why won't he go to the doctor?": The psychology of men's help seeking. *International Journal of Men's Health, 2*(2), 93–109.

Massoglia, M., & Remster, B. (2019). Linkages between incarceration and health. *Public Health Reports, 134*(1_suppl), 8S–14S. https://doi.org/10.1177/0033354919826563

Mejia, X. E. (2005). Gender matters: Working with adult male survivors of trauma. *Journal of Counseling & Development, 83*, 29–40.

Miller, N. A., & Najavits, L. M. (2012). Creating trauma-informed correctional care: A balance of goals and environment. *European Journal of Psychotraumatology, 3*, 17246. https://doi.org/10.3402/ejpt.v3i0.17246

Montague, B. T., Rosen, D. L., Solomon, L., et al. (2012). Tracking linkage to HIV care for former prisoners: A public health priority. *Virulence, 3*(3), 319–324.

Morrison, J. A. (2012). Masculinity moderates the relationship between symptoms of PTSD and cardiac-related health behaviours in male veterans. *Psychology of Men & Masculinity, 13*, 158–165.

National Research Council. (2012). *Reforming juvenile justice: A developmental approach.* The National Academies Press.

Needels, K., Stapulonis, R. A., Kovac, M. D., et al. (2004). *The evaluation of health link: The community reintegration model to reduce substance abuse among jail inmates: Technical report.* Mathematica Policy Research.

Nurse, A. M., Sankofa, J., Cox, A., et al. (2018). Juvenile corrections in the era of reform: A meta-synthesis of qualitative studies. *International Journal of Offender Therapy and Comparative Criminology, 62*(7), 1763–1786. https://doi.org/10.1177/0306624X17727075

Quam, S., et al. (2020). Racial identity, masculinities, and violence exposure: Perspectives from male adolescents in marginalized neighborhoods. *Journal of Adolescent Health, 67*(5), 638–644. https://pubmed.ncbi.nlm.nih.gov/32943288/

Ragonese, C., Shand, T., & Barker, G. (2019). *Masculine norms and Men's health: Making the connections.* Promundo-US.

Rich, J. D., Wohl, D. A., Beckwith, C. G., et al. (2011). HIV-related research in correctional populations: Now is the time. *Current HIV/AIDS Reports, 8*(4), 288–296.

Robertson, S. (2007). *Understanding men and health: Masculinities, identity, and Well-being.* Open University Press.

Sandman, D., Simantov, E., An, C., et al. (2000). *Out of touch: American men and the health care system.* Commonwealth Fund New York.

Schnittker, J., & John, A. (2007). Enduring stigma: The long-term effects of incarceration on health. *Journal of Health and Social Behavior, 48*(2), 115–130.

Shields, D. M. (2016). Military masculinity, movies, and the DSM: Narratives of institutionally (en)gendered trauma. *Psychology of Men & Masculinity, 17*, 64–73.

Smiler, A. (2004). Thirty years after the discovery of gender: Psychological concepts and measures of masculinity. *Sex Roles, 50*(1–2), 15–26.

Snyder, H. N., & Sickmund, M. (2006). *Juvenile offenders and victims: 2006 national report.* Office of Juvenile Justice and Delinquency Prevention.

Van Der Kolk, B. (2014). *The body keeps the score: Mind, brain and body in the transformation of trauma.* Penguin UK.

Vaswani, N., Cesaroni, C., & Maycock, M. (2021). Incarcerated young men and boys: Trauma, masculinity and the need for trauma-informed, gender-sensitive correctional care. In A. Cox & L. S. Abrams (Eds.), *The Palgrave international handbook of youth imprisonment. Palgrave studies in prisons and penology.* Palgrave Macmillan. https://doi.org/10.1007/978-3-030-68759-5_17

Wade, D., Varker, T., Kartal, D., et al. (2016). Gender difference in outcomes following trauma-focused interventions for posttraumatic stress disorder: Systematic review and meta-analysis. *Psychological Trauma, 8*, 356–364.

Wang, E. A., Hong, C. S., Shavit, S., et al. (2012). Engaging individuals recently released from prison into primary care: A randomized trial. *American Journal of Public Health, 102*(9), e22–e29. https://doi.org/10.2105/AJPH.2012.300894

Welfare, H. R., & Hollin, C. R. (2015). Childhood and offense-related trauma in young people imprisoned in England and Wales for murder and other acts of serious violence: A descriptive study. *Journal of Aggression, Maltreatment & Trauma, 24*, 955–969.

Chapter 15
Conclusion: Future Directions in Global Health Promotion with Young Men of Colour

Derek M. Griffith, James A. Smith, and Daphne C. Watkins

Introduction

We have assembled more than a dozen chapters written by scholars worldwide in this book. The chapters describe insights and strategies to promote the health and wellbeing of boys and young men of colour (BYMoC) in our efforts to close the "know-do" gap (Bacchi, 2008) – and to achieve men's health equity (Griffith et al., 2019a, b). A key component of closing the "know-do" gap is building from the global literature on men's health and masculinities and not simply from the literature that critiques men, the role of hegemonic masculinity, and power relations between men and women (Robertson & Kilvington-Dowd, 2019).

Despite the variations across geography, topic, and developmental period for BYMoC described in the chapters of this book, overall this volume serves as a preliminary look at the types of health promotion programs and approaches being pursued with BYMoC worldwide, and that also require our attention. This corpus

D. M. Griffith
Department of Health Management and Policy, School of Health, and Center for Men's Health Equity, Racial Justice Institute, Georgetown University, Washington, DC, USA
e-mail: Derek.Griffith@georgetown.edu

J. A. Smith (✉)
Rural and Remote Health, College of Medicine and Public Health, Flinders University, Darwin, Northern Territory, Australia

Menzies School of Health Research, Charles Darwin University, Darwin, NT, Australia
e-mail: james.smith@flinders.edu.au

D. C. Watkins
School of Social Work, University of Michigan–Ann Arbor, Ann Arbor, MI, USA
e-mail: daphnew@umich.edu

© Menzies School of Health Research, the rights holder, and The Editor(s) (if applicable) and The Author(s), under exclusive license to Springer Nature Switzerland AG 2023
J. A. Smith et al. (eds.), *Health Promotion with Adolescent Boys and Young Men of Colour*, https://doi.org/10.1007/978-3-031-22174-3_15

of scholarship provides illustrative examples of health promotion efforts with Indigenous BYMoC in Australia, Canada, and New Zealand, and Black American and Latinx BYMoC from the United States. Future editions of this book should expand on what we have highlighted by highlighting health promotion programs that demonstrate the kind of work being done with and in service of BYMoC in Asia, Africa, and the Caribbean, not to mention BYMoC from other countries. Because all our chapters reflect health promotion scholarship from high-income countries, it will be imperative to include scholarship and health promotion models from low- and middle-income countries.

Another significant gap in the literature is a thorough examination of promising strategies to promote the health and wellbeing of BYMoC who identify as gay, bisexual, transgender, queer, and questioning. This is an essential area of scholarship in the health promotion of BYMoC that, regrettably, does not receive the attention it deserves. Namely, for gay, bisexual, transgender, queer, and questioning BYMoC, their sexual and gender identity and sexual orientation may be particularly fundamental to how they see themselves and how others see and interact with them. Therefore, future editions of this book should include chapters that speak to the unique experiences of BYMoC across various sexual and gender identities. Furthermore, future editions of this book should also underscore a more nuanced analysis of promising health promotion approaches with BYMoC living in rural and remote contexts, as deeper examinations of their unique experiences are also warranted.

By anchoring health promotion strategies in the history and lived experience of BYMoC, the authors highlight the importance of considering the regional, national, and local contexts that shape masculinities and determinants of health that intersect with gender ideals in this critical period in the life course (Lohan, 2007; Watkins, 2012). These approaches to operationalising masculinities as the foundation for promoting the health, mental health, and wellbeing of BYMoC avoid the pitfalls that men's health scholars have eschewed, such as not celebrating multiple masculinities (i.e., masculinities vs. masculinity); reducing masculinities to characteristics of the individual; framing masculinities mainly as a proxy for a "deficit" view of men in relation to their health and wellbeing practices; and not recognising that masculinities are socially contingent and diverse (Robertson et al., 2016). Thus, one of the high costs of focusing primarily on hegemonic masculinity rather than masculinities is that we miss how masculinities are negotiated in everyday life and the social, cultural, and other contextual forces forming the nuances around the development of health promotion efforts (McVittie et al., 2017). Nonetheless, it is critical to note that young men who have particularly restrictive ideas about masculinities and manhood are more likely to bully, harass, binge drink, have traffic accidents, meet criteria for depression, and consider suicide (Heilman et al., 2017). Thus, attention to masculinities and our efforts to promote health and wellbeing among BYMoC should be viewed not as a niche interest, but as a costly factor adversely affecting our economies and societies (Heilman et al., 2017) in the short- and the long-term.

The chapter authors in our book provide a range of examples demonstrating how health promotion efforts for BYMoC and other men can be grounded in the historical, social, political, and cultural roots and contemporary determinants of masculinities, health, and wellbeing (Robertson et al., 2016). Building on the foundation laid by Robertson et al. (2016) and others, models, frameworks, and lessons learned from the scholarship collected in this book highlight the importance of recognising how heterogeneous BYMoC are in different social contexts. They also demonstrate why diversity is critical to building health promotion efforts that represent and resonate with BYMoC in ways that are consistent with their efforts to "do" gender (McVittie et al., 2017).

While not explicitly named or cited by the chapter authors, the notion of masculinities and gender identities being shaped and performed in communities of practice (Creighton & Oliffe, 2010) is a common theme throughout the book. Creighton & Oliffe's framework is helpful for examining and illustrating how males are defined by age, psychosocial development, and the sociocultural identities that have been politically mobilised to define the lenses through which we view their shared experience as BYMoC. Creighton and Oliffe (2010) discuss the importance of this theoretical framework for investigating and understanding how men's identities are learned and reproduced within racial, ethnic, and cultural subgroups and locations and masculinities. These chapters highlight the importance of understanding the shared network of people that define BYMoC's identities and the norms and practices that shape what it means to be part of those communities that are consistent with this theoretical framework (Creighton & Oliffe, 2010).

Another theme of the book involves the complexity that 15-to-24-year-old males grapple with in moving from adolescence to adulthood. Adulthood is a social construction that has real consequences for how BYMoC conceptualise, prioritise, and ideally promote health and wellbeing during a phase of life that is difficult to define and challenging to navigate (Griffith et al., 2019a, b). There is no professional agreement on the age range or definition of young adulthood. Consequently, health promotion interventions for young adults are often grouped with adolescents (Cunningham & White, 2019). BYMoC have expectations for how they see themselves when they reach certain ages or developmental milestones (e.g., formal schooling), make key decisions regarding progeny and partnerships status, and accept or are given specific roles in their families or communities. Despite this, the expectations of others in their social networks or communities of practice may change. These personal and social expectations can have important implications for the health and wellbeing of BYMoC and their motivation and ability to participate in programmatic health promotion efforts. For example, the support that many BYMoC have enjoyed through boyhood and adolescence dissipates or may be actively withdrawn when others view them as young adults (Cunningham & White, 2019).

In sum, we affirm that BYMoC are an important subgroup of males to study and the chapters of this book support our affirmation. We are honoured to have compiled such important efforts to promote the health and wellbeing of BYMoC for this book. We thank our colleagues for working with us to disseminate such outstanding scholarship and, most importantly, for doing the kind of work that will impact BYMoC throughout their lives. The contributing authors' chapters demonstrate the complexity of masculinities, multiple determinants of health and well-being, and strategies that promote the health and wellbeing of BYMoC. We hope this work educates, inspires, and stimulates new models, interventions, collaborations, and research that helps BYMoC realise their health, well-being, and life goals.

References

Bacchi, C. (2008). The politics of research management: Reflections on the gap between what we 'know' (about SDH) and what we do. *Health Sociology Review, 17(2), 165–176.*

Creighton, G., & Oliffe, J. L. (2010). Theorising masculinities and men's health: A brief history with a view to practice [report]. *Health Sociology Review, 19*(4), 409–418.

Cunningham, M., & White, A. (2019). Young adulthood and health disparities in African American males. In D. Griffith, M. Bruce, & R. Thorpe (Eds.), *Men's health equity: A handbook* (pp. 57–71). Routledge.

Griffith, D. M., Bruce, M. A., & Thorpe, R. J., Jr. (2019a). Introduction. In D. Griffith, M. Bruce, & R. Thorpe (Eds.), *Men's health equity: A handbook*. Routledge.

Griffith, D. M., Jaeger, E. C., Sherman, L. D., & Moore, H. J. (2019b). Middle-aged men's health. In D. Griffith, M. Bruce, & R. Thorpe (Eds.), *Men's health equity: A handbook* (pp. 57–71). Routledge.

Heilman, B., Barker, G., & Harrison, A. (2017). *The man box: A study on being a young man in the US, UK, and Mexico.* Promundo-US.

Lohan, M. (2007). How might we understand men's health better? Integrating explanations from critical studies on men and inequalities in health. *Social Science & Medicine, 65*(3), 493–504. https://doi.org/10.1016/j.socscimed.2007.04.020

McVittie, C., Hepworth, J., & Goodall, K. (2017). Masculinities and health: Whose identities, whose constructions? In *The Psychology of Gender and Health* (pp. 119–141). Elsevier.

Robertson, S., & Kilvington-Dowd, L. (2019). Masculinity and men's health disparities: Conceptual and theoretical challenges. In D. Griffith, M. Bruce, & R. Thorpe (Eds.), *Men's health equity: A handbook* (pp. 10–24). Routledge.

Robertson, S., Williams, B., & Oliffe, J. (2016). The case for retaining a focus on "masculinities" in men's health research. *International Journal of Men's Health, 15*(1), 52–67.

Watkins, D. C. (2012). Depression over the adult life course for African American men: Toward a framework for research and practice. *American Journal of Men's Health, 6*(3), 194–210.

Index

Printed in the United States
by Baker & Taylor Publisher Services